Javier Salazar
Edith Castellanos C
Claudia B Enriquez H

Knowledge of contraceptive methods in young Mexicans

Javier Salazar
Edith Castellanos C
Claudia B Enriquez H

Knowledge of contraceptive methods in young Mexicans

Knowledge of contraceptive methods in adolescents of the Telebachillerato El Nigromante, Veracruz

ScienciaScripts

Imprint

Cover image: www.ingimage.com

This book is a translation from the original published under ISBN 978-620-0-03309-3.

Publisher:
Sciencia Scripts
is a trademark of
Dodo Books Indian Ocean Ltd. and OmniScriptum S.R.L publishing group

120 High Road, East Finchley, London, N2 9ED, United Kingdom
Str. Armeneasca 28/1, office 1, Chisinau MD-2012, Republic of Moldova, Europe
Printed at: see last page
ISBN: 978-620-7-00943-5

Table of Contents :

Knowledge of contraceptive methods in young Mexicans

Knowledge of contraceptive methods in adolescents of the Telebachillerato El Nigromante, Veracruz.

Dr. Javier Salazar Mendoza
Dr. Edith Castellanos Contreras
Dr. Claudia Beatriz Enriquez Hernandez

Knowledge of contraceptive methods in adolescents of the Telebachillerato El Nigromante, Veracruz.

Gabriela Berenice Cuervo Pablo

Authors

Castellanos Contreras Edith

Bachelor's Degree in Nursing, Master's Degree in Nursing Sciences and Doctorate in Legal, Administrative and Educational Sciences. Full-time Professor "C", in the Faculty of Nursing Veracruz of the Universidad Veracruzana, with Recognition of the Desirable Profile PRODEP; member of the Academic Body Human Development-Veracruz (UV-CA-275) and the Network of Academic Bodies and Researchers for Sustainable Human Development, Professor with recognition for Teaching Merit 2016, State Coordinator of the Master's Degree in Nursing at the Universidad Veracruzana (ecastellanos@uv.mx).

Enríquez Hernández Claudia Beatriz

Bachelor's Degree in Nursing, Master's Degree in Nursing Sciences and Doctorate in Occupational Health Sciences. Full Time Professor "C", with recognition to the Desirable Profile PRODEP; Leader of the Academic Body Human Development-Veracruz (UV-CA-275). Responsible to the Universidad Veracruzana of the networks: Human Development and Network of Nursing Academic Bodies of the Universidad Veracruzana and member of the Basic Academic Core of the Master's Degree in Nursing of the Faculty of Nursing Veracruz (beenriquez@uv.mx).

Salazar Mendoza Javier

Bachelor in Nursing, Master in Nursing and Doctor in Legal, Administrative and Educational Sciences, collaborator of the Academic Body Human Development-Veracruz (UV-CA-275) and the Network of Academic Bodies and Researchers for Sustainable Human Development; Full-time Professor of the Faculty of Nursing Orizaba, Universidad Veracruzana, with recognition to the Teaching Merit 2018 and 2019, with recognition to the Desirable Profile PRODEP. Leader of the Academic Collaboration Group: nursing care, addictions and mental health and member of the Basic Academic Core of the Master's Degree in Nursing of the Faculty of Nursing Veracruz (jasalazar@uv.mx).

Co-authors

Cabrera Martínez Margarita

Bachelor's Degree in Nursing and Midwifery and Master's Degree in Nursing Sciences. Professor of the Faculty of Nursing Orizaba, Universidad Veracruzana, member of the Network of Academic and Research Bodies for Sustainable Human Development and the Academic Collaboration Group: nursing care, addictions and mental health. (margcabrera@uv.mx).

Carral Hernández Brenda

Bachelor's Degree in Nursing, Professor at the Universidad Veracruzana, Faculty of Nursing Veracruz, member of the Academic Body Human Development-Veracruz (UV-CA-275) and the Network of Academic and Research Bodies for Sustainable Human Development (bcarral@uv.mx).

Contreras Miranda María de Jesús

Bachelor's Degree in Nursing, Master's Degree in Nursing Sciences and Doctor in Public Administration and Government. Full-time Professor at the Faculty of Nursing Veracruz; member of the Academic Body Human Development-Veracruz (UV-CA-275) and the Network of Academic Bodies and Researchers for Sustainable Human Development and member of the Basic Academic Core of the Master's Degree in Nursing of the Faculty of Nursing Veracruz (jescontreras@uv.mx).

Conzatti Hernández María Esperanza

Bachelor's Degree in Nursing, Master's Degree in Nursing Sciences. Full-time Professor and Director of the Faculty of Nursing Orizaba, Universidad Veracruzana, member of the Network of Academic and Research Bodies for Sustainable Human Development and the Academic Collaboration Group: nursing care, addictions and mental health (econzatti@uv.mx).

Cuervo Pablo Gabriela Berenice

Student in Social Service, Bachelor's Degree in Nursing, Universidad Veracruzana, Faculty of Nursing, Veracruz. (berenice_cuervo@hotmail.com).

Fernández Blanca Flor

Bachelor's Degree in Nursing, Master's Degree in Educational Research and PhD in Education. Full-time Professor "C", with recognition to the Desirable Profile PRODEP; member of the Academic Body Human Development-Veracruz (UV-CA-275) and the Network of Academic Bodies and Researchers for Sustainable Human Development. Professor with recognition for Teaching Merit 2011; coordinator of Research in the Faculty of Attachment and member of the Basic Academic Core of the Master's Degree in Nursing of the Faculty of Nursing Veracruz (blfernandez@uv.mx).

Gonzalez Angulo Pedro

Bachelor in Nursing and Master in Nursing, collaborator of the Academic Body Human Development-Veracruz with key UV-CA-275 and the Network of Academic Bodies and Researchers for Sustainable Human Development; Full-time Professor at the Universidad Juárez Autónoma de Tabasco, in charge of the Educational Program of the Bachelor's Degree in Nursing of the Multidisciplinary Academic Division of Jalpa de Méndez. Representative of the Nursing and Health research group with PRODEP profile (petga82@hotmail.com).

González Riego Roberto Alejandro

Bachelor's Degree in Psychology and Master's Degree in Business Administration in the area of Human Resources at Tecnológico Milenio. Professor of the Faculty of Psychology at the Universidad Veracruzana; collaborator of the Cuerpo AcadémicoDesarrolloHumanoVeracruz (UV-CA-275),(robergonzalez@uv.mx).

Méndez Cordero Ernestina

Bachelor's Degree in Nursing and Pedagogy. Specialist in Surgical Nursing, Higher Education, Administration and Teaching, Master in Education, Doctor in Education and Doctor in Public Administration and Government, former Director of Nursing UMAE, IMSS, Full Time Professor "C" and member of the Basic Academic Core of the Master in Nursing of the Faculty of Nursing Veracruz, Universidad Veracruzana, with recognition to the Desirable Profile (PRODEP), Member of the Advisory Council of Linkage, recognition of teaching merit 2019, collaborator in the Academic Body Human Development (UV-CA-275) and the network of Academic Bodies and researchers for Sustainable Human Development (ermendez@uv.mx).

López Ocampo Miguel Ángel

Bachelor in Nursing, Master in Nursing, Professor of the Faculty of Nursing Veracruz, collaborator of the Academic Body Human Development Veracruz (UV-CA-275), and the Network of Academic Bodies and Researchers for Sustainable Human Development (milopez@uv.mx).

López Posadas Jesús Radai

Bachelor's Degree in Nursing from the Universidad Veracruzana, School of Nursing Orizaba, member of the Network of Academic and Research Bodies for Sustainable Human Development and member of the Association of Researchers for Sustainable Human Development (radalpz@gmail.com).

López Mora Gloria

Bachelor's Degree in Nursing, Master's Degree in Nursing Sciences and Doctor in Public Administration and Government. Full-time Professor at the Veracruz School of Nursing, Universidad Veracruzana; member of the Academic Body Human Development-Veracruz (UV-CA-275) and the Network of Academic Bodies and Researchers for Sustainable Human Development and member of the Basic Academic Core of the Master's Degree in Nursing of the Veracruz School of Nursing (glmora@uv.mx).

Rodríguez Muñoz Ivett

Bachelor in Nursing, Master in Educational Sciences and Master in Psychology and Community Development, Specialist in Community Psychology and Doctor in Education. Full-time Professor at the Faculty of Nursing Orizaba, Universidad Veracruzana; member of the Academic Collaboration Group Nursing care, addictions and mental health and the Network of Academic and Research Bodies for Sustainable Human Development (iverodriguez@uv.mx).

Summary

Introduction: the World Health Organization (2016), defines adolescence as the period of human growth and development that occurs after childhood and before adulthood, between the ages of 10 to 19 years and constitutes it as a stage of considerable risks and the social context influences it in a determined way.

Objective: To determine the level of knowledge of contraceptive methods in adolescents of the Telebachillerato El Nigromante, Veracruz.

Methodology: quantitative, descriptive, prospective and cross-sectional design, in 53 students from 15 to 21 years old, of high school level.

Results: 54.7% are female and 45.3% are male. **Conceptual dimensions:** 92.4% know that the use of contraceptives is intended for the entire sexually active population and 62.3% are aware that they prevent pregnancy and protect against sexually transmitted diseases.

Importance of their knowledge: 77.3% agree that in addition to protecting a pregnancy, they prevent the transmission of sexually transmitted infections, 83% affirm that condoms are the only way to protect against them.

Use of existing contraceptive methods: 41.5% of the students affirm that vasectomy and tubal ligation are not permanent contraceptive methods, 22.7% do not identify the rhythm method.

Frequency of method use: 96% think that condoms should be used only once and are not reusable and 77.4% mention that condoms should be placed before initiating sexual intercourse for greater effectiveness, therefore, the general objective is answered that 76.5%, have high and medium knowledge (24.5%), of contraceptive methods, coinciding with Aranda et al. (2017), and Jimenez (2016), contrasting with Sanchez et al. (2015), Vargas et al. (2016) and Moreno and Rangel (2012), since their populations, obtained high knowledge.

Key words: knowledge, contraceptive methods, adolescents.

Chapter I

State concerned

ESS. Cuervo Pablo Gabriela Berenice
LE. López Posadas Jesús Radai ME. López Ocampo Miguel Ángel Mtro. González Riego Roberto Alejandro ME. González Angulo Pedro LE. Carral Hernández Brenda

Introduction

Contraceptive methods (MAC) are procedures that prevent pregnancy in sexually active women, whether they or their partners use them. They can be hormonal or non-hormonal, transitory or definitive, technology-based or behavioral. The health professional should inform about all the options and verify the eligibility criteria, in such a way as to facilitate the user to make a free and informed decision. It can also provide guidance on the management of side effects, or possible problems that arise, and offer to change the MAC, if the user so desires (ICMER, 2018).

On the other hand, the World Health Organization (WHO) defines adolescence as the period of human growth and development that occurs after childhood and before adulthood, between 10 and 19 years of age. It is one of the most important transitional stages in human life, characterized by an accelerated pace of growth and change (WHO, 2009).

Adolescence, likewise, is a period of preparation for adulthood during which a number of important developmental experiences occur. Beyond physical and sexual maturation, these experiences include the transition to social and economic independence, the development of identity, the acquisition of the skills necessary to establish adult relationships and assume adult roles, and the capacity for abstract reasoning. Although adolescence is synonymous with exceptional growth and great potential, it is also a time of considerable risk, during which the social context can have a determining influence (WHO, 2009).

The main interest of the study Knowledge of contraceptive methods in adolescents of the Telebachillerato El Nigromante, Veracruz is to check if the knowledge of the students of the school is high or low, in addition to determine whether or not they infer or not the sociodemographic data. Hoping to obtain positive results from this study and, if not, to be able to make interventions to improve the levels obtained. For this purpose, an instrument was applied, with which the necessary information was collected in order to carry out the research work.

It is made up of five chapters, where the first one describes and poses the problem to be studied, as well as the research question: what is the knowledge of contraceptive methods that adolescents have. It also presents the general and specific objectives of the project: to determine sociodemographic data, to know the concepts they have about the subject, to identify the most commonly used methods and to classify the importance of using contraceptives.

In the reference framework, studies related to the topic of this study are presented in order to compare the results obtained in different years and places, and also to broaden the topic of study by presenting information on knowledge of contraceptive methods.

Chapter IV covers everything related to the study, such as the population to which the instrument was applied, the material used, the description of the procedure to be used, and the results obtained after analyzing the data collected.

The results are represented by descriptive data through the use of statistical tests that prove the proposed hypotheses. After this, the results obtained are discussed theoretically with other investigations, giving the conclusion for future studies. Finally, the bibliographical references that supported the construction of the project and the annexes that were useful for carrying it out are presented.

Description and problem statement

According to data from the National Institute of Statistics and Geography (2016), one in six births occurs in young people between the ages of 15 and 19, a regrettable fact, as this situation could be prevented with the regular use of contraceptives that are easy to obtain and ingest, in addition to offering high effectiveness.

Also, in the newspaper Excelsior (quoted by Silva, 2013), it was noted that the national coordinator of the Young People Program of the Mexican Foundation for Family Planning indicated that the early initiation of sexual relations and the lack of use of contraceptive methods are the most important factors in the increase of unplanned or unwanted pregnancies in adolescence.

Similarly, there are data showing that 1.5% of adolescents did not use any contraceptive method in their first sexual encounter, so it is essential for young people to have regular counseling, as a visit to a health specialist is essential to ensure access to effective fertility control (Silva, 2013).

The use of family planning methods is a responsible activity that aims to avoid risky sexual behavior, the spread of Sexually Transmitted Infections (STIs) or the genesis of an unwanted pregnancy, situations that are of great importance for public health, therefore it is necessary to know the level of knowledge, practices and attitudes of young people about sexuality, in order to design education and communication strategies that develop healthy behaviors (Mosquera & Mateus, 2003). It is true that adolescence undergoes rapid and profound changes that mark each individual in a different way. In spite of this, it is commonly considered as a healthy subset of the population, thus downplaying the importance of their health needs.

The World Health Organization (WHO, 2014) in its report Health for the world's adolescents, depression is the leading cause of illness and disability among young men and women between the ages of 10 and 19. Adolescents as a vulnerable population have a series of problems that start from different origins, such as alcohol consumption, drugs or bullying, body image disorders, eating disorders, depression, emotional disturbances, unwanted pregnancies and STI contagion.

It is important to bear in mind that the onset of active sexual life in adolescents is not predictable, since this event usually happens unexpectedly, thus leading to a lack of preparation and the use of a contraceptive method.

In Mexico, adolescents start this process earlier and earlier, often before the age of 15. The newspaper Excélsior (cited by the Ministry of Public Education, 2015), reveals that young people in high school had their first sexual encounter between the ages of 12 and 15.

From this, it can be deduced that four out of ten high school students began their active sexual life in high school, the seriousness of this situation is that a quarter of them did not use a contraceptive method to avoid sexually transmitted infections or an unplanned pregnancy, this increases by 37% the possibility of academic dropout at the high school level (SEP, 2015). It is said that the average age to start an active sexual life is at 15 years old, statistics from SEP, revealed that four out of ten adolescents had their first sexual intercourse at 12, 13, 14 or 15 years old, but more than 50% of them, do not know the correct use of contraceptives. According to a survey by the Latin American Center for Health and Women (SEP, 2015), this lack of knowledge causes four out of ten pregnancies to occur in girls aged 12 and 15.

In that same year, the SEP reinforced actions to prevent early pregnancy, since this can affect the educational progress of young people; for this reason, information must be provided in schools to avoid them. They also applied a survey on Exclusion, Intolerance and Violence in High Schools, which shows that 40% of males and 29% of females begin their sexual life in high school, a similar percentage to those who did so in secondary school.

Therefore, it is necessary to carry out this project in order to determine and identify the true level of knowledge that young people from El Nigromante high school have, as well as to determine where they have more weaknesses in the subject and take advantage of these areas of opportunity.

On the other hand, this problem is very common nowadays, as more and more adolescents are having sex at an early age and it is impossible to prevent young people from becoming sexually active in middle or high school, so they need to acquire clear and open information that gives them the possibility to make responsible decisions.

This study will serve to determine the knowledge that adolescents have about contraceptive methods and thus make some recommendations and carry them out with the study population. It is expected to be able to implement teaching strategies in the students, reinforcing the knowledge that was classified with low percentages.

Likewise, the study aims to benefit nursing students and teachers, since, by knowing the results, they will be able to evaluate strengths and weaknesses, improve in terms of dimensions with lower percentages and implement actions that favor them.

The present research will be a way of evaluating the students of the campus, determining the proposed objectives and, in this way, verifying the hypothesis or hypotheses proposed. In addition, continuing to conduct studies in the population will help to have a follow-up and check whether or not there is progress with the strategies implemented.

Research question

Based on the problems presented above, various search sources were consulted: books, printed and electronic journals, databases, scientific articles, and world, national and state registries, and the following research question was posed:

What is the knowledge of contraceptive methods that adolescents from Telebachillerato El Nigromante, Veracruz have?

Objectives

General

To determine the level of knowledge of contraceptive methods in adolescents of the Telebachillerato El Nigromante, Veracruz.

Specific

Characterize the sociodemographic data of the population.

To evaluate the students' concept of contraceptive methods.

To identify the contraceptive methods of greatest selection and use in the study population.

To classify the knowledge and importance of contraceptive methods in adolescents of the Telebachillerato.

Hypothesis

H_1. The level of knowledge of contraceptive methods among adolescents in the Telebachillerato El Nigromante, Veracruz, is low because sociodemographic characteristics are involved.

H_0: The level of knowledge of contraceptive methods among adolescents in the Telebachillerato El Nigromante, Veracruz, is high because sociodemographic characteristics do not play a role.

Variables

Independent

Teenagers from Telebachillerato El Nigromante, Veracruz.

Dependents

Knowledge of contraceptive methods.

Operationalization of Variables

Variable	Definition	Indicators	Instrument
Adolescents of the Telebachillerato El Nigromante, Veracruz	Persons who have completed basic education and are enrolled in a Telebachillerato school belonging to a rural community, with indistinct socio-demographic characteristics, in order to obtain the certificate of higher secondary education.	• Age • Marital status • Religion • Sex • Semester in progress • Number of siblings • Place between siblings • They have a scholarship • Average	- Data identification card 9 items
Knowledge of contraceptive methods	Information stored with experience or acquired formally, in health centers, school or with health professionals, regarding contraceptive methods, including use, frequency, recommendations and risks of malpractice.	- Concept - Importance - Type and frequency	- Level of Knowledge about Contraceptive Methods s (Aranda, Hualopa, Vicentr & Millones, 2017). 21 items

Chapter II

Basis of reference

Dr. Fernández Blanca Flor
ME. Gonzalez Angulo Pedro
Enríquez Hernández Claudia Beatriz ESS. Cuervo Pablo Gabriela Berenice Dr. Méndez Cordero Ernestina LE. López Posadas Jesús Radai **Referential Framework**

In the first place, the origin of knowledge from a philosophical point of view begins with Socrates, who was a Greek philosopher considered one of the greatest, Plato's teacher, who had Aristotle as a disciple; all three are representatives of Greek philosophy. Plato (427 B.C-347 B.C), expresses that "knowledge is the inherent possession of truth, an understanding of reality without having learned of it through sensory experience", evidence of this is the notion of "truth", the division between "doxa" (opinion) and "episteme" (science).

On the other hand, Aristotle (384 B.C.-322 B.C.) mentions that "knowledge is obtained through the senses, that is, through experience and contact with nature". Philosophy, religion and science were in disagreement.

With Christianity the idyll ended and there was a rupture, in view of this, St. Augustine said that one cannot be a Christian and a philosopher at the same time "because the pretension of mind in arriving at truth is vain, saying: truth is arrived at only by revelation through faith", he affirmed that time and the universe arose at the same time. In the Middle Ages, the birth of some kind of knowledge outside religious dogmas was not accepted, a fact that explains the way in which science was catapulted.

After that, in the modern age there were changes and innovation, scientific knowledge represented a fundamental pillar within the revolution, because it inspired progress and the use of the scientific method, which encouraged development, new ideas emerged in most areas. Positivism, union of all sciences, makes hierarchy as mentioned by Auguste Compte (1788-1857). Another important personality was Pierre Duhem (1861-1916), who describes knowledge as fallible and with the obligation to check whether it is false or true.

At present there are multiple points related to knowledge, defining it as a process developed by man to learn his world and realize himself as an individual. In the search for knowledge there was a long way to go, from Platonic ideas to reasoning, in order to understand the processes around them, to find an answer to each thing or fact that arises (Semilla, 2011; Marcos, 1998; Hoffe, 2003).

At the same time, the Descriptors in Health Sciences (DeCS, 2018), mention that knowledge is a body of truths or facts accumulated in the course of time, the sum of information collected, its volume and nature, in any civilization, period or country.

The term knowledge, is used in the sense of fact, information and concept; but also as understanding and analysis; the human species progresses to the extent that it accumulates experiences of other generations and manages to systematize them (Casaya, 2017).

However, there are different types, in relation to empirical or vulgar knowledge, by the observation of man is located in reality, in conjunction with knowing is granted curiosity and experiments with their senses, this learned from everyday life, is called empirical, since it derives from experience and any human being has it.

On the other hand, scientific knowledge is when man seeks a breakthrough to understand the circumstance he explores and obtain these. Research is employed and its aim is to explain every thing or fact that happens around him to determine both laws or principles that govern his world.

When talking about the knowledge that exists in Mexico in relation to the use of contraceptive methods, in the first place, the young female population between 15 and 24 years old, 97.4% expressed knowing at least one method of family planning in 2009, this proportion increased with respect to 1987, which was 91.5%.

On the other hand, adolescent fertility continues to be unplanned and there is an increase in sexually transmitted diseases, and the young population, despite having knowledge, is unable to accept the use of a contraceptive method in sexual relations. In spite of knowing about the existence of family planning methods, it should be asked whether adolescents have access to them and, once they do, whether they know the proper way to use them.

Even so, there is a socially disadvantaged population, this phenomenon is marked by factors such as a lower level of academic training, with 61.9% of young people with no schooling compared to 99.1% who have high school and above. Adolescents and rural youth with 92.0% to 98.9%. Finally, those women aged 15 to 24 years who speak an indigenous language with 79.7% versus 98.3% young people who do not speak their native language. The most known contraceptive methods are modern with respect to the traditional ones in both rural and urban places, on the other hand, women living in the countryside present low levels of knowledge regarding condoms, IUDs and pills (CONAPO, 2014, CONAPO 2016).

Likewise, the information contained in the article conducted by Sánchez, Dávila and Ponce (2015), showed that adolescents had received knowledge of the usefulness of contraceptive methods, obtaining as the main source teachers (37.5%), followed by health personnel (31.7%), parents (21.7%), media (5.8%) and finally friends (3.3%).

Contraceptive methods have their history throughout time and have been modified up to the present time. Historical elements will be taken up again to know what types of MAC (Contraceptive Methods) were used to avoid conception and how many of them are still used today.

When approaching a little bit of history it can be mentioned that fertility control has been one of the great concerns of people since ancient times and they have developed different ways to avoid conception, for example: douching, amulets, barriers, coitus interruptus, use of acid fruits or combinations of different herbs, all these types of methods were used to avoid unwanted pregnancy.

The history of contraception began to be written 6 million years ago, emerging at the precise moment when the hominid female decided to make her sexual desire independent of her menstrual cycle, establishing an enormous difference with the rest of the animal species that existed on earth (Martos, 2009).

It is known that nomadic tribes already used some forms of natural contraception to prevent pregnancy, and it has been reported that some mummies discovered in ancient Egypt had small rounded stones, pieces of ivory or bones inserted into the uterus (Sanyo & Molina, 2005).

On the other hand, it is essential to mention the Papyrus Ebers, the oldest book of medical treatises written in ancient Egypt, which describes a plug of gum Arabic and dates that served as a spermaticide and this happened in 1550 BC. Similarly, it has been documented that in the period between 1550 and 1850 BC vaginal washings with honey and sodium bicarbonate are described to prevent pregnancy (Lopez, 2003).

By the period 2000 B.C. the use of a small cone made of pomegranate seeds and wax had been documented, this method was invented by the Egyptians to prevent ovulation and is recognized as the first contraceptive with natural estrogens, however, in the world there were more harmful practices with little foundation, for example, in China women took mercury to prevent pregnancy.

Around the year 70 BC, there was a doctor named Soranos Ephesus who was the most important gynecologist of antiquity and one of the first to issue recommendations aimed at preventing pregnancy, he said that when the man was about to ejaculate, the woman should hold her breath, then get up, squat down and try to sneeze and drink something cold. Another strange custom existed in the 8th century, the Persians believed that sneezing and doing the seven magic jumps backwards after intercourse would dislodge the semen from the vagina.

Ten centuries later, in the eighteenth century, in France, every good hotel had a postcoital douche available to its guests, in the belief that vaginal douching was a good contraceptive method, but, even today, in the twenty-first century, these beliefs still exist (Ayala & Pereira, 2014).

In Greece and Rome, people used animal bladders and intestines as condoms to prevent the passage of semen into the uterine cavity, thus preventing the spread of venereal diseases. Breastfeeding was also known to have some degree of efficacy as a secondary natural contraceptive (Sanyo & Molina, 2005).

Martos (2009), mentions coitus interruptus as one of the most widely used contraceptive methods to avoid pregnancy, since it did not require potions or washing, it only required the man to withdraw from the vagina before ejaculating and thus the objective was achieved, and today its practice is still very popular.

Later in the nineteenth century, vaginal douches appeared as contraceptive method, a process that consisted in that after sexual intercourse, women were washed in the vagina, using soap, lemon or vinegar, or even a combination of the three materials.

By the 20th century, scientific studies demonstrated that hormones control the menstrual cycle in women and that the brain and ovaries are involved in their production. Lopez (2003) mentions that by the 1920s, a German laboratory investigated these sexual glandular products and manufactured the first cyclic preparation and years later American researchers discovered that estrogen inhibits the ovulation process.

In the 60's the first contraceptive pill was approved, giving a great step forward to female sexuality, simultaneously the condom began to be manufactured with latex, demonstrating that when used correctly and systematically, it is effective against pregnancy and is safe for almost everyone, except for people who are allergic to the manufacturing material, although few individuals have this reaction (Lopez, 2003).

The male condom has been shown to be the only contraceptive method that protects against the transmission of almost all Sexually Transmitted Diseases (STDs) and includes a high degree of protection against Human Immunodeficiency Virus (HIV). However, transmission of STDs is still possible if there are genital lesions outside the area that is covered with latex (Sanyo & Molina, 2005).

Zipper in 1967, designed the well-known "T" with copper, a plastic device in the shape of a T in whose vertical arm is wound a spiral of this metal. But it was not until 1970 when Scomegna demonstrated that by adding steroids and specifically progesterone to the horizontal branch of the T, a contraceptive effect was achieved, notably reducing menstrual loss and dysmenorrhea.

This same year, the Intrauterine Device (IUD) began to be manufactured, these were medicated or bioactive with copper ions, silver or hormones, increasing contraceptive efficacy and reducing side effects (Sanyo & Molina, 2005). As for definitive methods, bilateral tubal obstruction (BTO) or salpingoclasia and vasectomy, they began in 1880 when Lungren performed the first surgical sterilization procedure on a woman.

Since then, more than 100 different techniques have been described for the definitive sterilization of females. As for vasectomy, it began in 1930 with Sharp, but it was in 1963 that Poffenberger published excellent results on this process (Sanyo & Molina, 2005).

When approaching this perspective from a national perspective, it is essential to mention that contraceptive methods are defined by the Official Mexican Standard for Family Planning Services (DOF, 1993), as those used to regulate the reproductive capacity of an individual or a couple in order to avoid unwanted pregnancies. Depending on the possibility of regaining fertility, they are classified as temporary or permanent.

Temporary contraceptives include the following: Oral hormonals which are divided into two groups, combined estrogen and progestin, those containing only progestin. Injectable hormonal contraceptives, which are long-acting temporary methods and are divided into two groups: combined estrogen-progestin and progestin-only contraceptives.

Subdermal hormonal, long-acting temporary methods, which are inserted subdermally and consist of a continuous and gradual release system of a synthetic progestin and do not contain estrogen.

Intrauterine devices are devices that are placed inside the uterine cavity for hormonal contraceptive purposes. There are also barrier devices and spermicides, characterized by preventing conception mechanically or chemically and their use is temporary.

On the other hand, it is worth mentioning the natural or periodic abstinence, these are used to control your reproductive capacity, they are based on the knowledge of the physiological events that occur during a normal menstrual cycle.

And among the permanent contraceptive methods are the following: bilateral tubal occlusion, is a permanent contraceptive method in women, which consists of the obstruction of both uterine tubes in order to prevent fertilization. Vasectomy, a permanent contraceptive method in men, which consists of bilateral occlusion of the vas deferens, in order to prevent the passage of sperm.

The Mexican Institute of Social Security (IMSS, 2015) defines contraceptive methods as a procedure performed to prevent fertilization or conception during sexual intercourse. The fundamental purpose of these is to prevent an unwanted pregnancy by preventing sperm from coming into contact with the egg and fertilization from occurring.

In relation to the legal aspects in Mexico, it is essential to cite the Political Constitution of the United Mexican States of 1917, article 4° states in the first, second and fourth paragraphs that men and women are equal before the law, in addition to being protected with respect to the organization and development of the family. It also states that everyone has the right to decide freely, responsibly and in an informed manner on the number and spacing of their children. In addition, every individual has the right to health protection.

The law will define the bases and modalities for access to health services and will establish the concurrence of the Federation and the federative entities in matters of general health (DOF, 2018).

On the other hand, the General Population Law, in Article 3, mentions in the second paragraph that the Ministry of the Interior will dictate and execute or in its case will promote before the competent agencies or corresponding entities, the necessary measures to: carry out family planning programs through educational services, public health with those available to the public sector, oversee that such programs and those carried out by private organizations, are carried out with absolute respect for the fundamental rights of man and preserve the dignity of families (DOF, 2018).

Likewise, the General Health Law, in Title Three "Provision of Health Services", Chapter V "Family Planning Services", includes the following articles: 67 family planning is a priority, and its activities should include information and educational guidance for adolescents and young people (Ministry of Health, 2005).

Likewise, to reduce reproductive risk, women and men should be informed about the inconvenience of pregnancy before the age of 20 or after the age of 35, as well as the convenience of spacing pregnancies and reducing their number; all this, through correct contraceptive information, which should be timely, effective and complete for the couple.

Article 68 states that family planning services include: the promotion of the development of educational communication programs on family planning services and sex education, based on the contents and strategies established by the National Population Council; the care and monitoring of those accepting and using family planning services.

The advisory for the provision of family planning services by the public, social and private sectors, and the supervision and evaluation of their execution, in accordance with the policies established by the National Population Council. The support and promotion of research on contraception, human infertility, family planning and human reproductive biology.

Participation in the establishment of suitable mechanisms for the determination, elaboration, acquisition, storage and distribution of medicines and other supplies for family planning services, collection, systematization and updating of the information necessary for the adequate monitoring of the activities developed (Ministry of Health, 2014).

Likewise, the Law for the Protection of the Rights of Children and Adolescents, in Title Two, "On the Rights of Children and Adolescents", Chapter Five "On the right to be protected in their integrity, freedom, and against mistreatment and sexual abuse", Article 21, first paragraph, states: "Children and adolescents have the right to be protected against acts or omissions that may affect their physical or mental health, their normal development or their right to education in the terms established in Article 3 of the Constitution".

Likewise, from the eighth chapter "On the Right to Health", Article 28, sections B, G and H are taken up again, since they are in accordance with what is proposed in this research: Article 28. Federal, Federal District, state and municipal authorities, within the scope of their respective competencies, shall coordinate in order to:

B. Ensure medical and sanitary assistance for the prevention, treatment and rehabilitation of their health. G. To pay special attention to endemic and epidemic diseases, sexually transmitted diseases and HIV/AIDS, promoting prevention and information programs about them. H. Establish measures to prevent early pregnancies (DOF, 2000).

On the other hand, the Official Mexican Standard, NOM 005-SSA2-1993, on Family Planning Services in its general provisions establishes that the purpose of this legislation is based on the fact that the services of information, orientation, counseling, selection, prescription and application of contraceptives, identification and management of cases of sterility and infertility, as well as STD prevention and maternal and infant care, constitute a set of actions whose purpose is to contribute to the achievement of a state of complete physical, mental and social wellbeing and not only the absence of disease during the reproductive process and the exercise of sexuality, as well as to the wellbeing of the population (DOF, 1993).

Regarding the global epidemiological picture: according to Trends in Contraceptive Use Worldwide over the past five decades, contraceptive use has increased markedly, such that nearly two out of every three women married or in union globally in 2015 were using some form of protection against pregnancy. Growth in use was especially rapid in Asia and Latin America and the Caribbean, while it has increased at a much slower pace in several regions of sub-Saharan Africa.

Percentage-wise at the regional level, the proportion of women aged 15-49 years using any contraceptive method has increased minimally or stabilized between 2008 and 2015. In Africa, it went from 23.6% to 28.5%; in Asia, modern contraceptive use has increased slightly from 60.9% to 61.8%, and in Latin America and the Caribbean the percentage has remained at 66.7%.

The use of male contraceptive methods represents a relatively small proportion of the above-mentioned prevalence rates, being limited to condoms and sterilization (vasectomy). An estimated 214 million women of reproductive age in developing countries wish to postpone or stop childbearing, but do not use any modern contraceptive method (WHO, 2015). The main reasons lie in the limited choice of methods; limited access to contraception, particularly by young people, poorer segments of the population or unmarried people; fear of side effects, sometimes suffered previously; opposition for cultural or religious reasons; poor quality services; mistakes at the beginning of using them and gender-barrier providers (WHO, 2018).

Unmet need for contraception remains high. This inequity is driven by a growing population and a shortage of family planning services. In Africa, 24.2% of women of reproductive age have an unmet need for modern contraceptives. In Asia, Latin America and the Caribbean regions where contraceptive prevalence is relatively high, unmet need accounts for 10.2% and 10.7%, respectively (United Nations Department of Economic and Social Affairs, 2015).

According to the National Survey of Demographic Dynamics (ENADID), 62.3% of young women between 15 and 29 years of age have initiated their sexual life; of these, one out of two (49.9%) did not use a contraceptive method during their first sexual intercourse. Differentiating by age group, for adolescents aged 15 to 19 years, one in three (29.2%) have already initiated their sexual life and of them, 44.9% declared not having used any contraceptive method during their first encounter (INEGI, 2015, CONAPO, 2014). On the other hand, 72.4% of young women aged 20 to 24 years and 90.1% of those aged 25 to 29 years are sexually initiated and the percentage of those who did not use any method in their first relationship increases with respect to adolescents to 45.8%.

Regarding the use of contraceptive methods, one in two (50.1%) of women aged 15 to 29 years is a current user and 16.2% is a former user; of these, 73.0% are in a marital situation, 20.5% have never been in a union and 6.5% are ex-union.

In contrast, the largest proportion of young women who are not current users have a non-union marital status; 7.8% are never in union and 4.1% are ex-union. In total, 22.1% of unmarried young women aged 15-29 years do not use contraceptives; among the reasons are that 38.6% do not need it or are pregnant, 21.0% do not use it because they want to become pregnant, and 11.1% have or had side effects.

It is worth noting that, by state, the highest proportion of women of childbearing age who use contraceptive methods are located in: Chihuahua (59.3%), Baja California Sur (58.1%), Nayarit (57.7%), Colima (56.7%) and Baja California (56.2 percent). Meanwhile, Chiapas (40.4%), Oaxaca (42.8%), Michoacán de Ocampo (46.2%), Guanajuato (47.3%) and Guerrero (47.8%) are the cities with the lowest percentages in the use of preventive methods for pregnancy or STD (INEGI, 2015).

In this sense, the method most used by women of childbearing age, currently users, is bilateral tubal occlusion (BTO) used by 48.6%, followed by non-hormonal or barrier methods with 30.4%, 13.5% use hormonal methods, 4.8% use traditional methods and 2.7% use vasectomy. It is worth noting that 78.2% of women between 45 and 49 years of age who use contraceptive methods report using BTO, while 66.9% of young women between 15 and 19 years of age report using non-hormonal methods.

This shows that there is a significant percentage of young people who do not use a contraceptive method despite their expressed desire to limit or space their offspring. According to the National Population Council (CONAPO, 2014), the unmet need for contraceptive methods for women of childbearing age in union was 4.9%. This percentage is higher for young women, 13.5% of adolescents are in this situation, while young women aged 20 to 24 and 25 to 29 years the unmet need is 9.8% and 6.6%, respectively (INEGI, 2016).

It should be noted that most of the data obtained on the use of contraceptive methods prefer to address them as contraception and focus on women, leaving aside men, from which it can be inferred that men are not interested in the use of the male condom, which is the only method that men can use, leaving a huge gap in statistical knowledge.

Regarding the state situation, given the importance of family planning in fertility decline, the National Survey of Demographic Dynamics obtained information on the knowledge and use of contraceptive methods among women aged 15 to 54.

The use of contraceptive methods in the State of Veracruz is low compared to the national level, 59.9% of the married or unmarried female population is a user of some method, while in the country as a whole the proportion reaches 63.1%.

The method most used by women in their first sexual intercourse is the condom; in this sense, adolescents are the ones who use it the most (90.3%). However, the response with the highest percentage for not using any method in Veracruz is that they did not know them (39.7%) compared to the rest of the republic (28.6%) (INEGI, 2016).

At the national level, the methods most familiar to the female population of reproductive age are pills (91.8%), female surgery (86.7%) and the intrauterine device (85.8%). In the state of Veracruz, out of every 100 women aged 15-49 years, 90 are familiar with pills, 88 with female surgery, 87 with IUDs, 83 with injections and 75 with condoms.

In 2014, the adolescent population showed an increase in the use of contraceptive methods with 62.7% compared to 2009 which was only 43.6%. On the other hand, male participation in contraceptive prevalence increased from 13.1% in 2009 to 15.6% in 2014. Although this figure increased, the figures do not exceed the national figures of 17.8% and 18.0%, respectively, however, despite the increase in contraceptive prevalence, it should be noted that it is precisely young people who have an unmet need with 11.6%, so work must be done to ensure access to and supply of contraceptive methods (INEGI, 2015).

Talking about the classification of oral hormonal temporaries, there are two components that give way to it, estrogens and progestin, obtaining three different presentations:

Those containing constant doses of estrogen and progestin in each tablet or tablet. They are presented in boxes of 21 drugs, some include seven additional tablets, which do not contain hormones, only iron or lactose, resulting in cycles of 28 tablets for administration without interruption. Those that include variable doses of estrogen and progestin, which are administered within the 21-day cycle, are called triphasic, because they include three different amounts of synthetic hormones (DOF, 1993).

Those 21-day packs contain 15 tablets with estrogen alone, followed by six with fixed doses of estrogen alone, plus some synthetic progestin, and are called sequential and should not be recommended for use as a contraceptive method.

Based on the form of administration, combined oral hormonal contraceptives, in the first treatment cycle, should preferably be initiated within the first five days of the menstrual cycle or, exceptionally, on the sixth or seventh day. In the latter case, a barrier method should be used simultaneously during the first seven days of the administration of the method (DOF, 1993).

In the presentation of 21 tablets, one tablet is ingested daily for 21 consecutive days, followed by seven days of rest, without medication. Subsequent cycles will begin at the conclusion of the suspension period of the previous cycle, regardless of when menstrual bleeding occurs.

In the presentation of 28 tablets, one tablet is ingested daily for 21 consecutive days, followed by seven days in which one tablet containing iron or lactose is consumed. Subsequent cycles begin at the end of the previous one, regardless of when menstrual bleeding occurs. This method should be suspended at the end of menstruation, two weeks before major elective surgery or during prolonged immobilization of a limb, to be restarted within the first five days of the menstrual cycle, as this may cause monthly disorders (DOF, 1993).

The contraceptive effectiveness of this method under normal conditions of use is 99%; however, the effectiveness can be reduced by up to 92% due to incorrect use. Some women may experience headache, nausea, vomiting, dizziness, mastalgia, chloasma and/or intermenstrual spotting.

On the other hand, progestin-only pills are offered in boxes containing 35 tablets or lozenges, and administration should preferably begin on the first day of the menstrual cycle. If such initiation takes place after the first and before the sixth day, it is necessary to supplement with a barrier method during the first seven days. One tablet is taken daily without interruption, even during menstruation.

Due to the shorter duration of its contraceptive effectiveness, it is necessary to take the tablet at the same time. In postpartum or post-cesarean section, when the woman is breastfeeding, it will be started after the sixth week; otherwise, after the third week. Upon complete cessation of lactation, a change to another contraceptive method may be recommended.

Under normal conditions of use, this method provides 90 to 97% contraceptive protection. However, it is limited to the day on which the tablet or dragee is ingested; if one or more are missed, the method is ineffective. Some women may experience menstrual irregularities (bleeding, prolonged spotting or amenorrhea), headache and/or mastalgia (DOF, 1993).

Now it is the turn to address injectable hormonal injectables, combined estrogen and progestin. There are four types: estradiol cypionate 5 mg + medroxyprogesterone acetate 25 mg in 0.5 ml of macrocrystalline aqueous suspension. Estradiol valerianate 5 mg + norestisterone enanthate 50 mg in 1 ml of oily solution. Estradiol enanthate 5 mg + dihydroxyprogesterone acetophenide 75 mg in 1 ml of aqueous suspension. Estradiol enanthate 10 mg + dihydroxyprogesterone acetophenide 150 mg in 1 ml of aqueous suspension.

It is administered by deep intramuscular route in the gluteal region. The initial application should be made within the first five days after the onset of menstruation. However, it can be started at any time, if it is reasonably certain that the user is not pregnant.

If the method is initiated after the fifth day of the menstrual cycle, a barrier method should be used simultaneously for the first seven days after the injection. Subsequent applications should be administered every 30 ± 3 days, regardless of when menstrual bleeding occurs.

Users of contraceptives and injectables that only contain progestin can switch to the combined injectable hormone, receiving the first application on the scheduled day of application.
Thereafter, it will be provided every 30 ± 3 days, regardless of when menstrual bleeding occurs (DOF, 1993).

These contraceptives should be discontinued 45 days before major elective surgery or during prolonged immobilization of a limb, and restarted two weeks later. Under usual conditions of use, this method provides greater than 99% protection and lasts up to 33 days after injection. However, an administration 33 days after the previous one does not guarantee protection.

Some of the side effects of this method include menstrual irregularities, headache, nausea, vomiting, dizziness, mastalgia and/or increased body weight (DOF, 1993).

For those containing only progestin, there are two presentations of injectable hormones: Norethisterone Enanthate (NET-EN), 200 mg, in ampoule with 1 ml of oily solution. Medroxyprogesterone acetate (DMPA), 150 mg, in ampoule with 3 ml of microcrystalline aqueous suspension. The form of administration is intramuscular. The initial application should be made in any of the first seven days after the beginning of the menstrual cycle.

Subsequent injections of DMPA should be given every three months and NET-EN every two months, regardless of when bleeding occurs. Under normal conditions of use, this method provides contraceptive protection greater than 99% (DOF, 1993).

The duration of contraceptive protection conferred by NET-EN extends to at least 60 days following injection, although it is generally longer, and for that conferred by DMPA, it ranges from 90 days immediately following injection, although it is generally longer. The use of these methods may cause menstrual irregularities, amenorrhea, headache, mastalgia and/or weight gain (DOF, 1993).

Norplant subdermal hormones consist of six dimethylpolysiloxane capsules, each containing 36 mg of levonorgestrel. Six drugs with individual dimensions of 34 mm in length by 2.4 mm in cross-sectional diameter, releasing on average 30 pg daily of levonorgestrel. The duration of the contraceptive effect is five years.

Implanon consists of an ethinylvinyl acetate (EVA) capsule containing 68 mg of etonogestrel. A rod 40 mm long by 2 mm in cross-sectional diameter releases an average of 40 pg of etonogestrel per day during the first year, in the subsequent 12 months, this release decreases to an average of 30 pg per day and in the third year an average release of 25 pg per day is estimated. The duration of the contraceptive effect is three years.

The method of administration is by insertion under the skin on the inner side of the arm, following the surgical norms and techniques recommended by the manufacturers. The insertion should preferably be performed within the first seven days of the menstrual cycle or on any other day, as long as it is certain that there is no pregnancy (DOF, 1993).

The removal of the implant should be done meticulously, being performed on established dates, to facilitate the procedure. It is convenient to locate the capsules manually before starting the procedure. The rods may be fragmented or break during the process. If the anatomical location of the implant is not certain, X-rays and/or ultrasound can be used. The same procedure is followed for the insertion, after asepsis, antisepsis and anesthesia.

The anesthesia should be infiltrated exactly below the implants, at their lower end. A small incision should be made, through which the capsule(s) should be removed one by one, starting with the most accessible ones. If it is not possible to remove all the implants, refer the user to a hospital unit to solve the problem (DOF, 1993).

Contraceptive effectiveness under normal conditions of use is over 99% during the first year. After that, it gradually decreases. The duration of protection is three to five years after insertion, depending on the type of implant.

Collateral side effects include hematomas in the area of application, local infection, dermatosis, menstrual irregularities (hemorrhage, prolonged spotting, or amenorrhea), headache, mastalgia and/or expulsion of the implant (DOF, 1993).

On the other hand, the intrauterine device (IUD) consists of a flexible polyethylene body, which contains an active ingredient or adjuvant that can be a copper and/or copper and silver filament or a deposit with a progestin. The presentation of this device is individual and is accompanied by an inserter, inside a sterilized package. It also has guide wires for its location and removal. The IUD can be inserted at the following times: intergestational period: it is preferably implanted during menstruation, or on any day of this cycle, when it is reasonably certain that there is no pregnancy (DOF, 1993). Post placenta: placement should be performed within 10 minutes after delivery of the placenta. This technique can be performed after delivery, or during a cesarean section.

Pre-discharge: after the resolution of any obstetric event at hospital discharge, placement is performed before the patient is sent home. Post-abortion: immediately after curettage or vacuum aspiration for abortion, at any age of pregnancy. Late Puerperium: between the fourth and sixth week post-abortion, post-partum and post-cesarean section.

Duration of contraceptive protection: varies according to the active ingredient or adjuvant they contain. The duration of effectiveness of type T Cu 380A devices is up to ten years and for Multiload 375 and 250 from three to five years. The same term applies to IUDs containing a progestin. At the end of the period of effectiveness of the IUD, if the user still requires this method, she should replace it with another, immediately after removal (DOF, 1993).

Contraceptive effectiveness: Under usual conditions of use, this method provides 95-99% protection. In general, the IUD is well tolerated by most users. Side effects are infrequent, generally limited to the first few months after insertion, and may manifest themselves as pelvic pain during the menstrual period and increased quantity and duration of bleeding (DOF, 1993).

Barrier condoms and spermicides: male condom. It is a device made of latex, closed at one end containing a receptacle to store the ejaculated semen and open on the opposite side which ends in a rim or border, it is applied to the erect penis during sexual intercourse to prevent the passage of sperm and microorganisms into the vagina. Some also contain spermicidal substances (nonoxynol-9).

This is the only method that contributes to the prevention of sexually transmitted infections, including HIV/AIDS. Its physical characteristics are: length: 170 mm (small), 180 mm (large), width: 49 mm (small), 53 mm (large), thickness: 0.05 to 0.08 mm.

How to use: a new condom should be used at each sexual intercourse and from the beginning of intercourse, each condom should be used only once, the date of manufacture should be verified, which should not be more than five years from its manufacture or the expiration date, is placed on the tip of the penis, before penetration and when erect, pressing the tip of the condom between the thumb and index finger, to avoid air bubbles and unrolling the penis in its entirety to the base.

When the man is not circumcised, he should retract the foreskin toward the base of the penis before inserting the condom. After ejaculation, the still erect penis should be withdrawn from the vagina, holding the condom at the base to avoid spilling semen or retaining it in the vaginal cavity. Knot the condom before discarding it to avoid spilling semen.

If necessary, only water-soluble lubricants should be used, never oil, to avoid loss of effectiveness of the condom. This method provides 85 to 97% contraceptive protection (DOF, 1993).

Female condom: is a transparent, soft and resistant sheath made of polyurethane, with two plastic rings, one at each end. The ring at the closed end is used to facilitate insertion and keep the condom attached to the cervix, the ring at the open end is wider and remains outside the vagina, covering the woman's genitals and the base of the penis. Broadens the range of contraceptive methods available, it is a good choice for many women and their partners. It protects the penis from contact with the vagina, prevents sperm from entering the cervical canal, and protects against sexually transmitted infections including HIV/AIDS.

This method provides contraceptive protection of 79 to 98% with correct and frequent use. The duration of contraceptive protection is limited mainly by the time of correct use of the method (DOF, 1994).

The female condom, like the male condom, is disposable and its usefulness is limited to a single coitus. There are no side effects from the use of condoms, but if they should occur, counseling should be reinforced and, if necessary, the method should be changed.

Spermicides: there are several presentations, some of which are: creams: the vehicle is stearic acid and derivatives, or glycerin. The spermicide is nonoxynol-9, or benzalkonium chloride. Eggs: The vehicle is cocoa butter, glycerin, stearin, or soap. The spermicide is benzalkonium chloride, nonoxynol-9, monoisoethylphenol polyethylene glycol, ether or polysulfuric acid polysaccharide ester. Aerosol foams: the vehicle is polyethylene glycol, glycerin or hydrocarbons and freon. The spermicide is nonoxynol-9, or benzalkonium chloride.

Form of administration: applied inside the vagina, 5 to 20 minutes before each coitus, if more than one hour passes before having another coital intercourse, a second dose of spermicide, either cream or foam, should be applied. If it is a tablet or suppository, it is introduced as deep as possible into the vagina (DOF, 1993).

Under normal conditions of use, this method provides contraceptive protection of 75 to 90% and its effectiveness can be increased by combining it with other barrier methods. The duration of contraceptive protection will depend on the type of product used, and will be limited to one hour, starting from the application of the spermicide in the vagina.

Natural or periodic abstinence methods: these require great motivation and participation of the couple, as well as the woman's ability to identify the physiological changes that occur during the month, in cervical mucus, basal temperature and other signs associated with the period of greatest probability of pregnancy or fertility (DOF, 1993).

In order for the practice of these methods to be most effective, couples must understand that the man is fertile all the time, while the woman is fertile only on certain days of the month. The calendar, rhythm or Ogino-Knaus method, as a result of observing a year's worth of menstrual cycles, the couple can estimate their fertile period, determined by subtracting 19 days from the shortest cycle, and 12 days from the longest cycle, during which time sexual intercourse should be avoided. Because few women have regular menstrual cycles, calculations of the fertile period are often too broad and require prolonged abstinence (DOF, 1993). The Temperature Method is based on a single sign, which is the elevation of basal body temperature.

The woman should measure her temperature in the morning, immediately upon waking up and before getting up or carrying out any activity, including eating or drinking, and at the same time after having slept for at least five continuous hours.

The measurement should always be made in the same place of the body (axillary region, mouth, rectum or vagina), however, the most accurate is the rectal route. A graphic record of the body temperature should be kept in order to recognize when ovulation occurred or not. This change is discrete, with a variation of 0.2 to 0.4 degrees Celsius, and should be recorded daily (DOF, 1993).

The cervical mucus or Billings method identifies the days of fertility and infertility using self-observation of cervical mucus during a menstrual cycle. To practice it, the woman must have the ability to establish the difference between dryness, moisture and increased moisture at the vaginal and vulvar level, this is only achieved through self-exploration, where a sample of cervical and vaginal mucus will be obtained to verify its appearance and elasticity.

Changes in the characteristics of cervical mucus are thought to occur during the menstrual cycle in response to the production of steroid hormones by the ovaries. The secretion of cervical mucus at the beginning of the menstrual cycle is scanty, with little or no filminess and is described as sticky, this phase is followed by an increase in estrogen concentrations, which give a sensation of wetness and a more abundant and lubricating cervical mucus, which is observed close to ovulation, and is characterized by increased wetness. The peak symptom, or cusp, is an elastic mucus, which, if taken between two fingers, is observed to be stringy (i.e., stretched or elongated like egg white) (DOF, 1993).

Sexual abstinence should begin on the first day of the menstrual cycle, when the abundant and lubricating mucus is observed, continuing until the fourth day after the peak date, when the maximum symptom or thinness of the cervical mucus is present.

In order to determine, with certainty, the manifestations related to the menstrual cycle, the dates of the beginning and end of menstruation, the days of dryness, of sticky or cloudy mucus, and of clear and elastic mucus should be recorded, according to the conventional symbology available for the method (DOF, 1993).

The last day of mucus secretion, called the peak day, is marked with an X and can only be confirmed until the following day, when the dryness returns, which determines the beginning of the infertile stage of the menstrual cycle, starting on the fourth day after the peak day.

The three days following the peak are marked 1, 2, 3; the last infertile days of the menstrual cycle are from the fourth day after the peak day to the end of the cycle.

When pregnancy prevention is desired, the couple should abstain from sexual intercourse: on all days when cervical mucus secretion is observed, until the fourth day after the peak day; on days of menstruation and on the day after any sexual intercourse, before the peak day (DOF, 1993).

The symptothermal method is so called because it combines various symptoms and signs with basal temperature, changes in cervical mucus and numerical calculation to determine the woman's fertile period. They can be associated with other changes, such as: abdominal pain associated with ovulation, intermenstrual bleeding, changes in the position, consistency, wetness and dilatation of the cervix, mastodynia, edema and mood changes.

Cyclic changes of the cervix occur more uniformly.

Acceptors of these methods can be trained by trained personnel. A long period of initial instruction and progressive counseling is required. The duration of contraceptive protection of natural methods depends on their constant and correct practice. No side effects attributable to these methods have been described. However, when there is a lack of collaboration between partners, this can be a cause of method failure and emotional stress (DOF, 1993).

Permanent methods: bilateral tubal occlusion is a definitive contraceptive method, which consists of bilateral occlusion of the uterine tubes. It provides contraceptive protection greater than 99%. However, the user should be warned of the probability of failure. The procedure is indicated for women of childbearing age, with an active sexual life, nulliparous, nulliparous or multiparous, who desire a permanent method of contraception, in the following conditions: satisfied parity, high reproductive risk, mental retardation. So far, there are no known side effects directly associated with the method. Occasionally, there may be problems associated with the anesthetic procedure (epidural block or general anesthesia), or surgical: (bleeding or infection), time of performance, the process can be performed in the intergestational interval, postpartum, transcesarean and postabortion (DOF, 1993).

Vasectomy is a permanent method of contraception for men, which consists of bilateral occlusion of the vas deferens, in order to prevent the passage of sperm. There are two procedures: the traditional technique (with scalpel) and the Li Shungiang technique (without scalpel).

Traditional technique with scalpel: surgical procedure, by which the vas deferens is ligated, sectioned or blocked, through two small incisions in the scrotum. No-scalpel Li technique: surgical procedure, by which the vas deferens is ligated and sectioned through a small puncture in the scrotal raphe.

In both techniques, electrofulguration can be used to block the vas deferens. This method provides contraceptive protection greater than 99%. No directly associated side effects are known to date. Occasionally, problems associated with the surgical procedure may occur: ecchymosis, surgical wound infection, granuloma, hematoma (DOF, 1993).

On the other hand, speaking of adolescents, it is necessary to point out that the population studied belongs to a rural community, therefore, according to the World Health Organization (WHO, 2016), the adolescent is the individual who goes through a stage of human life in which: biologically, the human being progresses from the initial appearance of secondary sexual characteristics to sexual maturity. Psychologically, the individual's mental processes and identification patterns evolve from those of a child to those of an adult, and socially, a transition is made from a state of total socioeconomic dependence to relative independence.

In relation to socioeconomic characteristics, the most important thing that happens to the adolescent, from the social point of view, is the intensity acquired by the relationship with his or her peer group. This group of belonging, using a language, clothing and ornaments different from those of adults, is fundamental for affirming their image and acquiring the security and/or social skills necessary for the future. There is also a critical review of the ethical and religious values learned in the family or at school. This is a necessary revision in order to incorporate these values as one's own and not imposed by others (DOF, 1993).

Adolescents have a great sense of justice, they defend it both individually and in the facts that affect humanity. They accept a punishment if they consider that it was deserved; but if they believe that it was unjust, they are provoked by a rebelliousness capable of not stopping until the previous mistake is corrected.

In such a case, the image of the authoritative adult loses respect and credibility. The family group falls into a conflict between rejection and dependence. The adolescent would like to be more independent, but the family ties, especially in the affective aspect, are very important.

Do not make the mistake of starting a competition between the family and the group of friends. Both the home and the group of friends are fundamental for adolescent development.

The family for unconditional emotional support throughout life and friends, as mentioned above, for the acquisition of the social skills that allow them to adequately incorporate themselves into the external world, the family being a protective system that does not provide sufficient knowledge in this area.

Finally, the discussion between rights and duties takes on significant importance. As they grow up, they acquire obligations and do not perceive the acquisition of new rights; this means that growing up is often lived with little enthusiasm. Complaining that adults are ambivalent in their dealings with them, illustrating it with the phrase: you are old enough to understand this, but still too young to do this other (Universidad de Chile, 2017).

According to the Asociación Mexicana de Agencias de Investigación y Opinión Pública A.C. (AMAI, 2004), for the classification of level 13 variables established by the Socioeconomic Levels Committee in August 1998 were defined.

The variables are the following: last year of studies of the head of household, number of light bulbs in the household, number of bedrooms excluding bathrooms, number of bathrooms with showers in the household, possession of cars (owned or not), water heater/boiler, type of floor (only cement or other material), vacuum cleaner, computer, microwave oven, clothes washer, toaster, and VCR.

With these 13 variables, six different socioeconomic levels were assigned, corresponding to the following classification: A/B: Upper Class-This is the segment with the highest standard of living. The profile of the head of household in these households is basically made up of individuals with a Bachelor's degree or higher. They live in luxury homes or apartments with all the amenities.

C+: Upper Middle Class, this segment includes those whose income and/or lifestyle is slightly above middle class. The profile of the head of household in these households is made up of individuals with a Bachelor's degree education. They generally live in their own homes or apartments, have some luxury and have all the amenities.

C: Middle Class, this segment contains what is typically referred to as the middle class. The profile of the head of household in these households is made up of individuals with a high school education. Households belonging to this classification are owned or rented houses or apartments with some amenities (AMAI, 2004).

D+: Lower Middle Class, this segment includes those households whose incomes and/or lifestyles are slightly lower than those of the middle class. This means that they are those who lead a better lifestyle within the lower class.

The profile of the head of household in these households is made up of individuals with a secondary or primary school education. The homes belonging to this segment are mostly owned by them, although some people rent the property and some are social housing.

D: Lower class, this is the middle segment of the lower classes. The profile of the head of household in these households is made up of individuals with an average primary school education (completed in most cases). The homes belonging to this segment are owned or rented (it is easy to find neighborhoods), which are mostly of social interest or of frozen rents.

E: Lower class is the lowest segment of the population. It is little included in the market segmentation. The profile of the head of household in these households is made up of individuals with a primary education level without completing it. These people do not own a place of their own and have to rent or use other resources to get one.

More than one generation usually lives in a single household and they are totally austere. The economic characteristics of an adolescent may vary according to the social class to which he or she belongs (AMAI, 2004).

In relation to personal characteristics. Adolescence is a time when emotions begin to come to the fore. Parents and teachers may observe argumentative and aggressive behaviors due to intense and sudden emotions. Adolescents are also regularly immersed in themselves. They care more about themselves because they are beginning to develop a sense of self, but they are also exploring their own thought processes and personality (Maier, 2017).

Possibilities begin to look endless during this stage, leading some teens to be overly idealistic. They also believe that their own thoughts and feelings are unique, doubting that others can possibly understand what they are going through.

For school characteristics. Academic performance in adolescence is the product of the interaction of a set of variables (known as conditioning factors of academic performance), which can be grouped following an ecological model, in 4 levels: personal factors (intellectual abilities, psychological and affective factors), family factors (educational level of parents, type of attachment with parents), school factors (inappropriate teaching methods, poor curriculum and scarce resources) and social factors (sociocultural environment, support networks) (Ruiz, 2013).

All these variables do not have the same weight within this multifactorial explanatory model. According to reports by the Organization for Economic Cooperation and Development (OECD, 2014), approximately 25% to 30% of the causes of school failure are not known. Between 5% and 6% of school success is due to the school climate, school policies, school resources and methodological aspects.

Therefore, it is possible to deduce that methodological changes, if not accompanied by other actions, will not obtain significant positive results. Almost 18% to 20% of school results are explained by the socioeconomic context of the school and its environment.

The psychological and affective characteristics of the student body account for almost 50% of the explanation of academic success. And how they interact in research using hypothetical causal relationship models, student aptitude only explains between 25% and 35% of the variance in academic achievement. Moreover, in correlational studies, between aptitude and achievement decreases as the learner moves up in grade level.

Effectiveness in learning is not only related to cognitive ability and aptitude, but also depends on how the adolescent uses that potential through personal learning styles, i.e., the different ways in which students perceive, structure, memorize, learn and solve school tasks and problems.

But, in addition to having skills and knowing how to use them to obtain satisfactory performance, it is also necessary to have what the student "already knows" (prior knowledge) in order to achieve truly meaningful learning. This prior knowledge is increasingly decisive as educational levels advance, and its absence ("lack of foundation") can make it impossible to understand future learning, especially in certain subjects (Ruiz, 2013).

On many occasions, there are adolescents who have sufficient intellectual capacity, however, they do not obtain good school results because they do not know what to do when faced with a given task, they fail to plan when trying to tackle it, they do not feel capable of solving it, or they do not choose the right strategy at the right time.

This means that, even if they have sufficient cognitive means and resources, because they do not know how to use appropriate learning strategies, consciously planning and controlling what they do, they do not achieve the expected results.

In order to learn, it is not only necessary to be able to do it and know how to do it, it is also necessary to have the necessary capabilities, knowledge, strategies and skills, that is, to have sufficient disposition, intention and motivation (affective-motivational variables), which allow the cognitive mechanisms to be set in motion in the direction of the objectives or goals to be achieved. Within the affective-motivational variables, causal attributions, achievement expectations, personal worth, self-efficacy and, above all, self-concept are included, since a reciprocal causal relationship has been found between academic self-concept and students' school experiences and/or achievements (Ruiz, 2013).

Weiner's motivational theory (1986) maintains that motivated behavior is a function of the expectations of achieving a goal and the value of that goal. According to this author, these two components are determined by the causal attributions expressed by personal beliefs about which causes are responsible for their successes or failures.

Weiner states that attributions are primary determinants of motivation, in that they influence expectations, affective reactions and, consequently, performance behavior and the results obtained. In the formation of self-concept and causal attributions, family socialization patterns are important. It is within the family bosom where the individual builds the basis of his personality, where he learns the first roles, models of conduct, begins to shape his self-image, learns the norms, the hierarchy of values that he will put into practice how to regulate himself. The family educational climate, which includes both the parents' attitude towards their children's studies and the affective family climate in which the child develops, together with the expectations they have placed in him/her, is the family variable that has the greatest weight in relation to school performance.

Variables that define parental involvement behaviors in their children's education have greater explanatory power than variables that define the characteristics of the family itself (Ruiz, 2013).

Of all these studies, parents' expectations of their children's ability to perform well academically is the variable with the greatest influence. It has a direct and positive influence on academic self-concept. That is, as parents' expectations about their children's ability increase, their self-concept increases and their self-confidence and academic motivation increase.

In addition, expectations of ability also have a positive impact on the processes of causal attribution of students' success or failure; thus, the higher the parents' expectations about their children's ability, the greater the tendency of their children to take responsibility for their positive academic achievements, and vice versa.

Contrary to popular belief, the rewards, external and contingent reinforcements for children's achievements, given by parents, do not favor academic achievement. It is found that the more they perform

This type of reinforcement is more detrimental to academic self-concept, decreases children's responsibility for achievement and the development of academic skills and, paradoxically, also results in lower student performance. Within the social variables, more and more importance is being given to the gender perspective.

Gabarro (2010), relates the differences in the prevalence of school failure by gender to the way women perceive the academic environment and the expectations they have in this context and their own social role. Different studies show that boys currently consider academics as something feminine, something that does not concern them and even humiliates them in their conquest of masculinity.

With regard to the epidemiology of adolescents, according to the Pan American Health Organization in 2007, it is defined as the stage between 10 and 19 years of age, this classification is based on the morbidity and mortality behavior of this population group. For operational purposes, it has been characterized into two subgroups: early adolescence from 10 to 14 years of age and late adolescence from 15 to 19 years of age.

By 2016 in Mexico there were 22,190,481 adolescents, this represents 20.63% of the total population. CONAPO estimates that by 2020 and 2050 the number of young people will decrease to 19.2 and 14.1 million people respectively. Despite the achievements during the last years, there are many problems and challenges that threaten the possibilities of healthy development of adolescents.

The health problems that appear most frequently are those of infectious origin, such as respiratory, gastrointestinal, urinary and sexually transmitted diseases; within the first twenty causes of medical attention, motor vehicle transportation accidents also appear.

Mortality: the adolescent population dies each year as a result of
The result of conditions that could have been prevented: mainly deaths caused by violence, either by direct action (homicides and suicides) or negligence (accidents).

Reproductive Health: Adolescents are the segment of the population most at risk for sexual and reproductive health problems, such as high rates of STI/HIV infection, unplanned pregnancies, and abortions. According to the 2005 National Youth Survey, most of those surveyed began sexual relations between the ages of 15 and 19. In the 2006 National Health and Nutrition Survey (ENSANUT), 14.4% of the country's adolescents reported having had sexual relations, the highest percentage being between 16 and 19 years of age with 29.6% of those surveyed (ENSANUT, 2006).

The prevalence of contraceptive use among women between 15 and 19 years of age who have initiated sexual relations increased from 36.4% in 1992 to 39.4% in 2006. Of all adolescents who have had sexual intercourse, it is observed that the percentage of use of some contraceptive method in the first sexual intercourse is higher in males. Of these, 71.5% reported having used some method, while in females the reported use was 44.2%.

The pregnancy rate in adolescents between the ages of 12 and 19 in 2005 was 79 pregnancies per 1,000 women. While the pregnancy rate among adolescents between 12 and

15 years of age was six pregnancies per 1,000, the number increased among 16 and 17 year olds to 101 pregnancies per 1,000, and the greatest increase was observed among 18 and 19 year olds, who reached a rate of 225 pregnancies per 1,000 women (ENSANUT, 2006).

Regarding the formation of the first union, 82.2% of the men and 65.8% of the women in the adolescent population declare themselves to be single. Likewise, 11.4% of them and 25.5% of them say they have married (Instituto Mexicano de la Juventud, 2006).

Related studies

In the thesis entitled Level of knowledge about contraceptive methods in adolescents of secondary education of the private educational institution Bertrand Russell, Los Olivos-2015 by Aranda, Hualpa, Vicente and Millones (2017), where they raised the main objective, to determine the level of knowledge that exists in the students of that institution.

The research was descriptive and its design, cross-sectional, which consists of the exploration and description of phenomena in real life situations. It offers a detailed description of the characteristics of certain individuals, situations or groups of 185 students between 11 and 18 years of age in secondary school, of which there are 99 males and 86 females.

The data collection technique used to obtain the information is the survey, the instrument used being the Survey of Level of Knowledge of Contraceptive Methods (ECMA), the name of the questionnaire, designed to identify the level of knowledge of high school students about contraceptive methods.

The instrument has the following aspects in its structure: it presents 21 questions on knowledge of contraceptive methods, divided into four dimensions: A. Concept: General according to WHO, B.
Importance: Of their knowledge, C. Type: Of contraceptive methods that exist and are used by MINSA, and D. Frequency: Of the use of the methods, according to MINSA. The general results obtained from the ECMA questionnaire show that "a high level of knowledge was found in 47.6% of the adolescents, followed by a medium level with 34.6% and a very low percentage of people with a low level of knowledge (17.8%).

The results obtained through the ECMA questionnaire with respect to the concept dimension show that the highest level of knowledge is medium with 51 .4%, followed by high with 47.6% and with a lower percentage of low level with 9.2%. This shows that the adolescents participating in the study are aware of what contraceptive methods are.

With respect to the dimension "importance", the highest number was found to be medium with 51.9%, followed by high with 45.4% and with the lowest percentage, low with 2.7%. It was found that adolescents have knowledge about contraceptive methods.

In the results obtained in the type dimension. It was found" that the highest percentage belonged to the medium level with 46.5%, followed by low with 34.1% and with a lower percentage of high with 19.5%. It was demonstrated", therefore, that a considerable part of the adolescent population surveyed has low level knowledge of the different contraceptive methods that exist.

Finally, in the type dimension, "medium level of knowledge was found in 56.2% of the students, followed by low level with 28.1% and with a lower percentage of high level with 15.7%.

It is evident that a considerable population of the surveyed adolescents does not have sufficient knowledge about the frequency with which contraceptive methods should be used in order to be effective.

In the research evaluation of knowledge and use of contraceptive methods in students of the high school N°2 of the City of Tulancingo de Bravo, Hidalgo 2015, by Vargas, Yunez and Ramirez (2016), with a cross-sectional approach in the period March to May 2016. A census was conducted in a general high school belonging to the Autonomous University of the State of Hidalgo, which is attended by adolescents from various municipalities in the region, highlighting that this institution is public and therefore is economically accessible, which allows young people from various socioeconomic levels to attend it.

The unit of observation: Students in computer science classes from 1st to 6th semester, of the 2,089 students invited to answer an online survey, 1,697 accepted, four surveys were eliminated because the participants were 20 years old or older and 15 because they answered less than 80% of the survey.

Regarding sociodemographic characteristics, of the 1,678 satisfactorily answered surveys, 58.34% were answered by women and 41.66% were answered by men (p=0.0000). The overall mean age was 16 years (p=0.0578). Fifty-four percent of the adolescents were found to be between 15 and 16 years of age; in relation to marital status, 98.69% were single and only 1.31% stated that they were in a union (p=0.0000).

In addition to studying, 18.12% also work and 71.87% mentioned living with both parents. According to the socioeconomic level, modified for this study according to the AMAI's 8x7 rule of 2011, 34.51% are reported with a high level, 35.52% with a medium level and 29.98% with a low level. At the time of the survey, the municipality where most of the students lived was Tulancingo with 64.18%, followed by the municipalities of Singuilucan with 11.1% and Cuautepec with 11%. Regarding the use of contraceptive methods in the last sexual intercourse, the highest proportion of use is found in men aged 15 to 16 years, in union, who in addition to studying work, who live with family members other than their parents and with a high socioeconomic level, which is the same proportion found in the use of MA in the first sexual intercourse, in addition women (RM=9.92), and men (RM=6.35), who use some MA in their first sexual intercourse, are more likely to use it in the last one, being statistically significant for both.

And the most used contraceptive methods in the first and last sexual intercourse were the male condom in addition to using the emergency pill as a second contraceptive method, both in men and women, it is noteworthy that in the last sexual intercourse the percentage of use for emergency hormonal as the condom is in men, but the use of another variety is in women, both in the first and in the second sexual intercourse.

Regarding the knowledge index, in general, a high average level was obtained , which tells us that adolescents have a good knowledge of contraceptive methods. Women between 15 and 16 years of age, single, living with both parents and with an average socioeconomic level were the ones with the greatest knowledge of contraceptive methods.

Jiménez, Vilchis and Martínez (2016), in their research Level of knowledge about contraceptive methods that students of a secondary school in Mexiquense have, posed the objective of analyzing the level of knowledge about contraceptive methods that students of a secondary school in Mexiquense have.

The focus of the study was quantitative, descriptive-cross-sectional, since data were collected at a specific time and date, in 646 students of the Juan Fernández Albarrán high school, with sampling: non-probabilistic at the discretion of the researcher and sample: 222 students of the afternoon shift, the inclusion criteria: students who had informed consent signed by their parents and assent signed by the parents themselves, using the data collection technique: survey.

Instrument: a questionnaire with 27 items was applied and validated by experts in the field. It was designed with closed questions; the first part covered the sociodemographic characteristics of the students, and the second part included questions related to knowledge of contraceptives, such as type and use.

Of the students surveyed, 51.8% were male, while 48.2% were female. The majority of the students surveyed were in the third year of secondary school with 45.9%, 38.2% of the second year students participated, while only 15.9% of the first year students participated.

Regarding the type of family, 68.8% are nuclear families, 19.4% are single-parent mothers, and 5.9% are single-parent fathers and extended families. In relation to the father's schooling, 46.5% studied up to secondary school, while 23.5% studied up to high school and only 14.1% have a higher level of education. With respect to the mother's schooling, 44.1% have a high school education, 30% have studied up to high school and only 7.6% have a higher level of education.

In relation to the knowledge of concepts about contraceptive methods it was found) that most students have general knowledge of the concepts, having that of the 9 questions the students had a maximum of 9 points and a minimum of 1, having as mean 5.7 and with ± 1.44.

Regarding the knowledge of the type of contraceptive methods, it was found that students had a maximum of 6 points and a minimum of 0, with a mean of 2.07 and ± 1.58, which indicates that most of the students do not know the types of contraceptive methods.

For the 1 knowledge of the use of contraceptive methods, it was found that of the 12 questions, the students had a maximum of 12 points and a minimum of 0, with a mean of 5.04 and ± 2.34, which shows that the students do not know how to use the different contraceptive methods.

According to the results obtained from the application of the questionnaire to the students of the Juan Fernández Albarrán secondary school, 64.7% have a medium level of knowledge about the topic, while 25.9% have a low level of knowledge and only 9.4% have a high level of knowledge. With the results of the percentages, we can say that Juan Fernández Albarrán secondary school students have deficient knowledge about contraceptive methods.

Sánchez, Dávila and Ponce (2015), in their article Knowledge and use of contraceptive methods among adolescents in a health center, with the aim of identifying the level of knowledge and use of contraceptive methods. The study was descriptive, observational and cross-sectional, non-probabilistic sample, sample size calculation for descriptive studies based on absolute difference criterion. The study was conducted in the health care services of the Ampliación Hidalgo health center, Tlalpan sanitary jurisdiction, of the Secretaría de Salud del Distrito Federal, Mexico, in the months of September and October 2014.

Adolescents aged 15 to 19 years with an active sexual life were included. After written informed consent, a questionnaire was administered with sociodemographic variables and questions to evaluate the use of contraceptive methods. The level of knowledge was classified according to the number of correct answers: null, low, medium and high; descriptive and inferential statistics were performed with the Mann-Whitney and Krusskall-Wallis U tests. Significance level 0.05, using the SPSS v 20 statistical program.

A total of 120 adolescents were included, with a mean age of 16.9 ± 1.3 years; 85 (70.8%) were female and 35 (29.2%) were male. The predominant marital status was single (73; 60.8%), followed by free union (40; 33.3%), and married (7; 5.8%). The mean number of years of study was 9.4 ± 1.3 years, with a minimum of 3 and a maximum of 15. The most frequent occupation was student (56; 46.7%); followed by home (33; 27.5%); student and employee (14; 11.7%); and employee and merchant (9.2% and 5%, respectively). The mean age of sexual debut was 15.10 ± 1.4 years, with a minimum of 11 and a maximum of 19 years.

Regarding contraceptive methods, the male condom was the most widely known (100%), followed by oral hormonal methods (87.5%) and the female condom (85.8%). Of the 120 adolescents, 117 (97.5%) had received information on how to use contraceptive methods; the most frequent sources of information were teachers (37.5%), followed by health personnel (31.7%). They concluded that it is important to improve the quality of education on knowledge and proper use of contraceptive methods, since most adolescents have a medium and low level of knowledge, which has an impact on their sexual and reproductive health.

However, it is important to provide quality care, with counseling and pre-registration of contraceptives in an easy and explicit manner, since most adolescents obtain contraceptives from commercial pharmacies, which generally do not take into account aspects such as acceptability, method safety and the characteristics of the adolescent in order to achieve better rates of use and continuity.

In the study Knowledge about contraceptive methods in 9th grade students of the Nuestra Señora de Lourdes School, Puerto Ordaz, Bolivar State, conducted by Moreno and Rangel (2012), they set out to determine the knowledge about contraceptive methods possessed by 9th grade students of the Nuestra Señora de Lourdes School in Puerto Ordaz, Bolivar State. A cross-sectional prospective descriptive study was designed.

The sample was represented by 100 students surveyed who obtained prior authorization from their representatives. The results showed that between the ages of 13 and 14 years old, 58.1% (43) had excellent knowledge, while 62.7% (54) of the female sex rated it as excellent.

Regarding the origin of the information, 45.0% (23) of the female sex and 44.8% of the male sex obtained the information through the media, while 42.9% (21) of the male sex and 39.2% (20) preferred to receive the information through the school. There were representative differences in the use of contraceptive methods in terms of sex: 90.2% (46) of the female sex do not use contraceptive methods, while 46.9% (23) of the male sex do use contraceptive methods.

It was concluded that the ninth grade students have excellent knowledge, evidenced in both dimensions, age and sex, with greater weight in ages 13-14 years and the female sex. It is recommended that students be informed about each of the contraceptive methods so that they can be alert and know the importance of using them and avoid possible consequences.

Definition of terms

Telebachillerato adolescents: young people who have completed basic education and are enrolled in a telebachillerato.

Menstrual cycle: period of 28 +/- 5 days between two menses during which ovarian follicle maturation, ovulation and formation of a corpus luteum take place (DOF, 1993).

Knowledge: set of information stored through experience or learning, or through introspection, (Pérez, 2008).

Informed consent: is the voluntary decision of the acceptor to undergo a contraceptive procedure, with full knowledge and understanding of the pertinent information and without pressure (DOF, 1993).

Contraindication: is the situation of health risk for which a contraceptive method should not be administered, applied or practiced (DOF, 1993).

Availability of contraceptive methods: users' certain possibility of obtaining contraceptive methods in the institutions of the National Health System or of acquiring them in pharmacies in the country (DOF, 1993).

Fertile or reproductive age: stage in the life of men and women during which they have the biological capacity to reproduce (DOF, 1993).

Contraceptive effectiveness: the ability of a contraceptive method to prevent pregnancy under the usual conditions of use, in a period of one year (DOF, 1993).

Sexually transmissible disease: infection acquired through sexual intercourse, exchange of sexual fluids or contact of genital mucous membranes (DOF, 1993).

Indication: prescription or application of a contraceptive method according to the needs, characteristics and health risk factors of the acceptor (DOF, 1993).

Exclusive breastfeeding: Feeding the newborn with breast milk, without the addition of other liquids or foods, avoiding the use of pacifiers or bottles (DOF, 1993).

Contraceptive methods: are those that prevent the viable birth of a new being, either by interfering with the normal mechanism of conception or, once pregnancy has occurred, by interrupting it (Aller & Pagés, 1998).

Family planning: the right of every person to decide freely, responsibly and in an informed manner on the number and spacing of their children and to obtain specialized information and appropriate services (DOF, 1993).

Precaution: is the situation of risk to health for which the convenience or not of administering, applying or practicing a contraceptive method should be evaluated under clinical criteria (DOF, 1993).

Sexual intercourse: for the purposes of this standard, only vaginal intercourse is considered sexual intercourse (DOF, 1993).

Reproductive risk: the probability that both the woman of childbearing age and her potential product will experience illness, injury or death in the event of pregnancy (DOF, 1993).

Reproductive health: is the state of complete physical, mental and social well-being and not only the absence of disease during the reproductive process, as well as in the exercise of sexuality (DOF, 1993).

Sexuality: set of anatomical, physiological and psychological-affective conditions that characterize each sex (Benetti, 2011).

Chapter III

Empirical basis

Dr. Contreras Miranda María de Jesús MCE. Conzatti Hernández María Esperanza ESS. Cuervo Pablo Gabriela Berenice Dr. Rodríguez Muñoz Ivett MCE. Cabrera Martínez Margarita Dr. López Mora Gloria

Nola Pender's theory of health promotion model

According to Mariner and Raile (2007), Pender was born in 1941 in Lansing, Michigan, United States and was the only child of parents who were staunch advocates of women's education. At the age of seven, she had the experience of watching her aunt receive nursing care, which created in her a great fascination for nursing work, her idea of the profession was caring and helping others to care for themselves.

Her family encouraged her in her goal of becoming a registered nurse, so she enrolled in nursing school at West Suburban Hospital in Oak Park, Illinois. She received her nursing degree in 1962 and began working in a medical-surgical unit in a Michigan hospital.

In 1964, Pender earned a Bachelor of Science in Nursing (BSN) from the University of Michigan. She earned a master's degree in human growth and development from Michigan State University in 1965, and a doctoral degree (PhD) in psychology and education in 1969 from Northwestern University in Evanston, Illinois. While earning her PhD, Pender experienced a shift in her thinking that led her to define the goal of nursing as the optimal health of the individual.

In 1975, Dr. Pender published a conceptual model of preventive health behavior, which formed a basis for studying how individuals make decisions about their own health care in the context of nursing.

In this article she identified factors that had influenced the decision making and actions of individuals to prevent disease (Mariner & Raile, 2007). In 1981, she was admitted as a member of the American Academy of Nursing and served as president in 1991 and 1993. In 1982, she presented the first edition of the health promotion model. In 1996, she presented the second edition of this model.

Nola J. Pender is recognized in the profession for her contribution with the Health Promotion Model. She proposed that promoting an optimal state of health was an objective that should take precedence over preventive actions. This was a novelty, since it pointed out the factors that had influenced the decisions and actions taken to prevent disease.

In addition, he identified that individuals' perceptual cognitive factors are modified by situational, personal, and interpersonal conditions, resulting in engagement in health-promoting behaviors when there is a pattern for action.

The Health Promotion Model (HPM), proposed by Pender (1998), is one of the most predominant in nursing science; according to it, the determinants that compose it (health promotion), and lifestyles, are divided into cognitive-perceptual factors, understood as those conceptions, beliefs or ideas that people have about health, which lead or induce them to certain behaviors or behaviors, which in this case, are related to decision making or health-promoting behaviors. The modification of these factors, and the motivation to perform such behavior, leads people to a highly positive state called health.

The conception of health, in Pender's perspective, starts from a highly positive, comprehensive and humanistic component, takes the person as an integral being, analyzes lifestyles, strengths, resilience, potentialities and capabilities of people in making decisions regarding their health and life.

This theory identifies preceptual cognitive factors in the individual that are modified by situational, personal and interpersonal characteristics, resulting in participation in health-promoting behaviors when there is a pattern for action.

The MPS serves to identify relevant concepts on health promotion behaviors and integrate research findings in such a way that facilitates the generation of testable hypotheses. In addition, it is based on educating people on how to take care of themselves and lead a healthy life (Mariner & Raile, 2007).

The meta paradigms, pointed out in the Health Promotion Model are: **health:** highly positive state and has more importance than any other general statement, **person:** individual and the center of the theorist, each one of them, is defined in a unique way by its own perceptual cognitive pattern and its variable factors, **environment:** it is not precisely described, but the interactions between the preceptual cognitive factors and the modifying factors that influence the appearance of health promoting behaviors are represented. **Nursing:** wellbeing as a nursing specialty, is responsible for health care, the basis of any reform plan for such individuals, the nurse is the main agent in charge of motivating users to maintain their personal health.

Nola J. Pender, proposed that promoting an optimal state of health was an objective that should take precedence over preventive actions. This was a novelty, as it identified the factors that had influenced the decisions and actions taken to prevent disease.

In order to analyze alcohol consumption in adolescents, from the professional nursing perspective, the Health Promotion Model (HPM), by Nola J. Pender (Pender, Walker, Sechrist, & Stromborg, 1998), which focuses on lifestyles and behaviors, directed at people in order to maximize their individual, organizational and community knowledge, is used.

Primary prevention focuses on people at risk for illness, secondary prevention focuses on those who have a diagnosed illness, however, both recognize that individuals have the capacity to self-direct change due to self-awareness and regulation, decision making and problem solving skills. The role of nursing is to promote a positive climate for change, serve as a catalyst for change, assist with various steps in the modification process, as well as increase the capacity of individuals to sustain change.

The use of theories and models of individual behavior are systematic attempts to explain why human beings do not engage in healthy behaviors and how they change negatively or implement new health attitudes (Pender et al., 1998).

The Model of Health Promotion (MPS), proposed by Nola J. Pender, undertakes lifestyles and behaviors in people whose purpose is to maximize their individual, organizational and community knowledge. Primary prevention focuses on people at risk of disease, secondary prevention focuses on subjects with diagnosed diseases.

Secondary prevention has a greater affluence of people with chronic degenerative diseases that continue with a worsening of the condition. In the case of primary prevention, this uses strategies that reduce or prolong the onset of the disease, such as diabetes, cardiac pathologies or cancer, while secondary prevention activities promote within the limits of the disease, when it is present (Pender, Walker, Stromborg & Sechrist, 2009).

Health promotion is an action that seeks to reduce or prevent a disease or condition and these, in turn, have had benefits in terms of quality of life and longevity.

Health promotion and primary prevention is based on behavioral or sociopolitical models of health care, which have shown different results in multiple health systems (Pender, 1998). People or individuals have the capacity to self-direct change due to self-awareness and regulation, decision making and problem solving abilities, the role of nursing is to promote a positive climate for change, serve as a catalyst for change, assist with various steps in the process of change, as well as increase people's capacity to sustain change.

The use of theories and models of health behavior, systematic attempts to explain why individuals do not engage in health behaviors and how they negatively change or implement new health attitudes (Pender, 1996).

It is understood that the mechanisms on behavior modification and sustainability of these changes are necessary to develop health promotion and prevention interventions, the MPS incorporates models and theories which are based on health and beliefs, the theory of reasoned action and the theory of self-efficacy and social cognitive theory.

Health personnel interventions can be directed at the individual's subjective beliefs and norms, whose individual influence will be assessed through outcomes that focus on individual perceptions of the normativity of other people's expectations and the motivation to meet the expectations that others expect (Pender, 1996).

The MPS of Nola J. Pender, is an attempt to represent the multidimensional nature of people, interacting with their intrapersonal and psychological environments, which are involved with health, in addition, it is integrated with three constructs and eleven concepts, taking up the theories: value of hope and social cognitive, within nursing with a holistic perspective of human function.

Individual characteristics and experiences are what each person maintains in a unique way, this being so, because of the effect of the actions, that is why it is important that the effect depends on the behavior and objective being considered.

The previous related behavior is proposed to obtain direct and indirect results with the possibility of influencing health promoting behavior, the direct effect of past behavior on current health promoting behavior due to habit formation, predisposed to obtain a behavior with certain specific attention and repetitive practice of the mentioned.

Personal factors predict a certain behavior given its form and the nature of the objective that is considered from the beginning and are categorized into biological, psychological and sociocultural. The specific cognitions and affect of the behavior, is the behavior considered as the most motivationally important, in these variables, the critical center is constituted, since they can be modified through interventions that ensure the effectiveness and efficacy of the behavioral change.

Figure 1 (Pender, 1998) shows the assessment of health beliefs, related to previous knowledge and experiences, determining the behaviors adopted by the person; according to the MPS proposed by Pender, they are given by:

Perceived benefits of action are the positive mental representations or reinforcement of the consequences of a behavior. Individual expectations is a coupling of a behavior that revolves around anticipatory benefits.

Perceived barriers to action are the unavailability, inconvenience, difficulty or time consumed in a particular action. Barriers are often seen as mental walls, obstacles and personal costs to undertaking a particular behavior.

The perception of self-efficacy is taken as a judgment of personal character with the ability to organize and carry out the course of action, it involves judgments that an individual has and can do with the skills he/she possesses.

The related affects of the activity consist of different components: emotional arousal, to act itself (related act), self-acting (self-relating), and the environment where the action is performed (related context). As a result, it is feeling a state that is likely to affect the individual and repeat the behavior again or maintain it for a prolonged time.

Personal influences, cognitions that involve the behavior, beliefs or attitudes of others, whether or not they correspond to reality. The primary source of personal influences on health promotion is family, peers and health care, including social norms, social support and modeling.

Situational influences refer to personal perceptions and cognitions about the situation or context that facilitates or impedes a behavior; in health-promoting behavior, these include perceptions and available options, demanding environmental characteristics (Pender, 1998).

The commitment to an action plan begins with a behavioral situation, which drives the individual into an action, unless they compete, demanding that it cannot be avoided. The MPS comprises an action plan that employs a fundamental monitoring process, creating a commitment to a specific time and place, in order to identify strategies that the person can choose, leading to the reinforcement of the behavior.

Competing demands and preferences at the time refer to behaviors that attempt to create awareness immediately, before health-promoting behavior planning is applied, creating a positive outcome in the individual in order to establish healthy lifestyles (Pender, 1996).

The behavioral outcome from the MPS is determined by the commitment to an action plan, which can be deviated by the immediate counter demands and preferences in each person, acting as a barrier to action, understood as anticipated, imagined or real blocks and personal costs of adopting a given behavior.

There are other barriers that can limit the adoption of a health behavior and are determined by the person in relation to the following (Pender, 1998): Age: particularly has to do to a large extent by a specific stage of the life cycle where the person is; from this stage on, lifestyle will be affected.

Gender: determinant of behavior, since being a man or a woman will cause the individual to adopt a certain posture regarding how to act, in addition to the prevalence of some diseases that will be reflected in a greater proportion in one of them.

Culture: is one of the most important conditions that lead people to adopt a lifestyle, whether healthy or not; it includes eating habits, leisure time, sports, among others.

Class or socioeconomic level: a fundamental factor when it comes to leading a healthy lifestyle, if you belong to the middle or high level, you will have more alternatives when choosing access to health care; while for a person with a low socioeconomic level, your options will be limited by the scarcity of economic resources, emotional states, self-esteem and degree of urbanization.

The commitment to an action is similar to the intention that each individual has, it is important to predict various health behaviors and to formulate specific strategies designed for the actions of a person, for this reason, it is of utmost importance that the Health Promotion Model be used to intervene in adolescents who have a recurrent consumption of alcohol, in order to impact their attitudes, knowledge and modification of lifestyles.

Figure 1
Health Promotion Model (Pender, 1998).

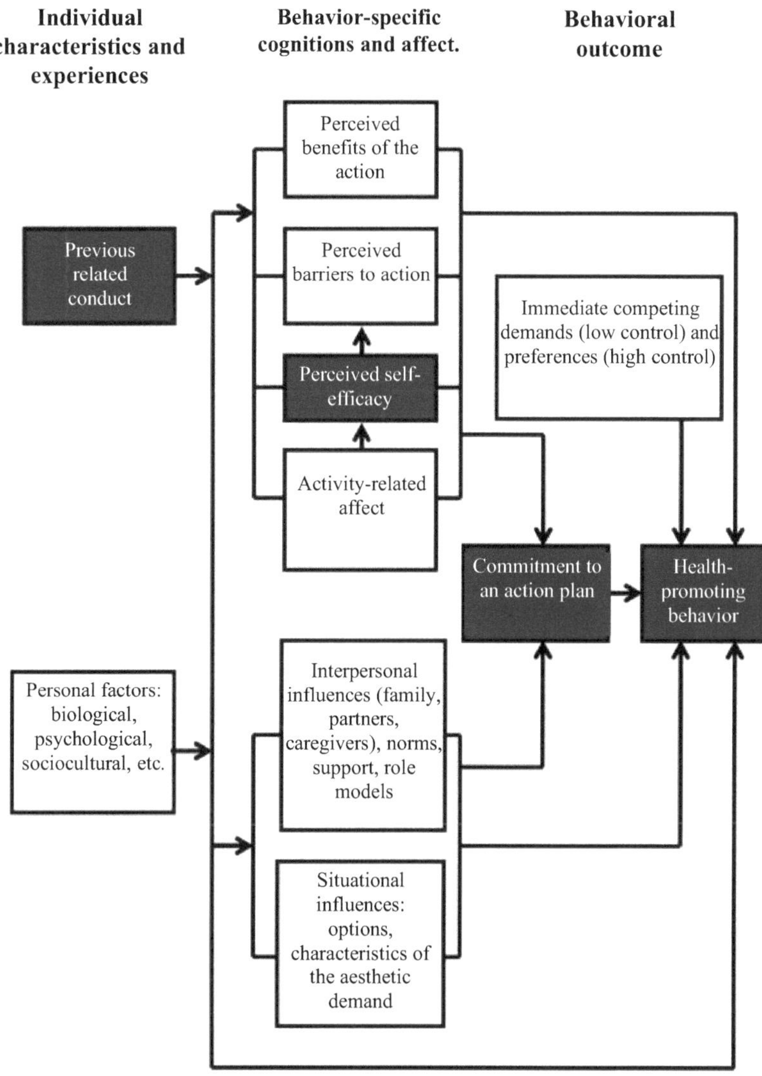

To address the problem of the level of knowledge of contraceptive methods, it was necessary to integrate the three constructs proposed by the Theory, and in turn, the key concepts that allowed to be the guide and support for the implementation of the study. Regarding individual characteristics and experiences, the concept of previous related behavior, cognitions and specific behavioral affect, perceived self-efficacy and behavioral outcome, commitment to an action plan, were taken to give way to Health Promoting Behavior (Figure 2).

The previous related behavior allowed us to assess the students' knowledge, frequency, importance and use of contraceptive methods. On the other hand, it was necessary to evaluate who informed them about this topic; therefore, it is necessary to point out that it was a young population.

A determining factor in obtaining truthful and assertive data was the authorization of the school's directors and the direct invitation to the participants to answer the instrument responsibly, ensuring the privacy of the data provided, as stipulated by the General Health Law, in the section on research with human beings (Secretaría de Gobernación, 2012), the Code of Nursing Ethics (CIE, 1953), and the Helsinki Declaration Standards (CONAMED, 2008).

The concept of perceived self-efficacy, from the construct: behavior-specific cognitions and affect, was evaluated in the participants, taking as a reference the importance for them, the knowledge of contraceptive methods taking into account age, culture, gender and religion, determinants of individual perception.

The above, showed a diagnostic overview, to reinforce the areas of knowledge and thus the modulation of behavior, through vocational training, allowing them to participate actively and effectively, personally, family and socially, identifying those points favorable to the high level of knowledge.

Regarding construct three: behavioral outcome; the concept of commitment to an action plan is similar to the intention of each individual to participate or not in the research study, therefore, the population in training was approached with the purpose of inducing them to participate in health care, highlighting the protective factors and the final result of modulating the behavior they currently perform.

Figure 2
MPS constructs and concepts used

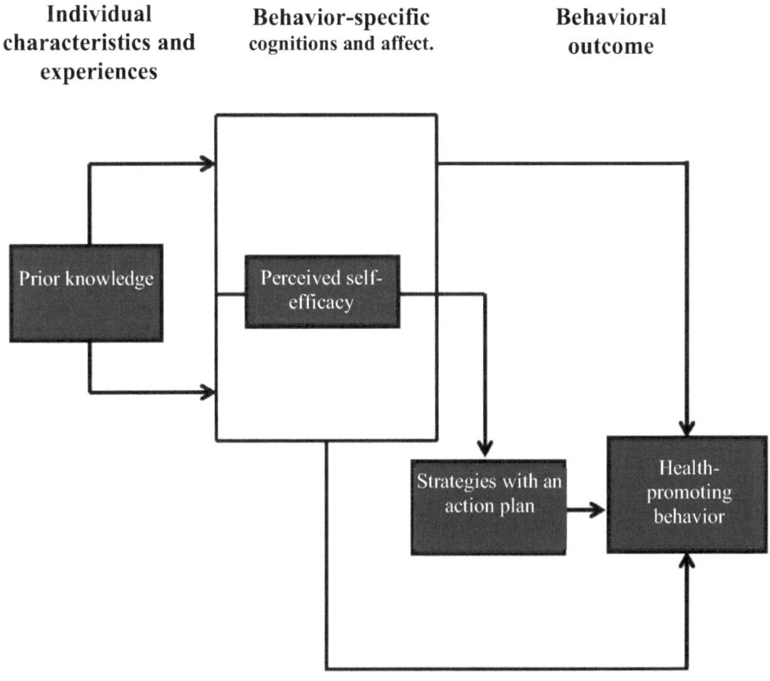

Chapter IV

Method of work

Dr. López Mora Gloria
Dr. Enríquez Hernández Claudia Beatriz Dr. Fernández Blanca Flor Mtro. González Riego Roberto Alejandro ESS. Cuervo Pablo Gabriela Berenice LE. López Posadas Jesús Radai **Type and design of the study**

This research, due to its structure, analysis and scope of the results is quantitative, of descriptive approach design or framework, in relation to the time of occurrence of facts and data recording is prospective and cross-sectional, according to the procedure for collecting information in a given period and the control that the researcher has of the variables in groups of individuals or units, detailing the knowledge of contraceptive methods that adolescents of the public Telebachillerato located in the community of Nigromante, in the state of Veracruz, have (Canales, Alvarado & Pineda 2013, Ortiz & García, 2014, Grove, Gray & Burns, 2016).

Population

The study was conducted in the Telebachillerato El Nigromante, Municipality of Playa Vicente, state of Veracruz, with a working universe of 53 students studying in the second, fourth and sixth semesters of the period August 2017-July 2018.

Sample design

For the purposes of the project, students in the second, fourth and sixth semesters of the Bachillerato Nigromante Veracruz were taken into account, obtaining a total of 53 students.

According to Polit and Hungler (2000), applying the formula with 95% statistical significance (Z=1.96), for finite populations and due to the number of people, it was decided to administer the instrument in the entire institution, representing 100%.

Sampling and sampling

To obtain the sample, the non-probabilistic convenience sampling method was applied, applying an instrument to the 53 students enrolled in the Telebachillerato El Nigromante, Municipality of Playa Vicente, in the state of Veracruz (Canales, Alvarado & Pineda 2013).

Selection criteria

Inclusion

Students aged 15 to 21 years from the Telebachillerato El Nigromante, Municipality of

Playa Vicente, in the state of Veracruz, with prior authorization from the institution's management staff to work with them, who signed the informed consent, enrolled in the second, fourth and sixth semesters, of the school period August 2017-July 2018, age, gender and religion indistinct, time availability and who agreed to participate, receive orientation and explanation of the project on the day the instrument was applied.

Exclusion

Students with any mental alteration, language and psychomotor problems were excluded, as well as pregnant women, as they are classified as a vulnerable population, according to the General Health Law in terms of research (Secretaría de Gobernación, 2012), and at risk for research studies (Tamayo, 2014).

Disposal

Persons who decided to abandon the research, omitted or answered a question twice, and those who left the instrument unfinished were eliminated.

Material

An identification form was used together with the instrument applied, where the sociodemographic data of each of the participants was obtained, i.e., age, sex, religion, current semester, whether they have any scholarship and, if so, the type of scholarship, as well as the number of siblings they have and the place they occupy.

In the second section , we present the Survey of Levels of Knowledge of Contraceptive Methods (ECMA), which assesses the variable under study, dividing it into four dimensions (concept, importance, type and frequency), elaborated by Aranda et al. (2017), consists of 21 items, indicating an existence of internal consistency, with a minimum score of 5 and a maximum of 21.

In order to obtain the reliability value of the ECMA, the authors conducted a pilot test at the El Paraíso Private Educational Institution with 46 students belonging to the 3rd and 4th grades of secondary school. Cronbach's Alpha was applied, obtaining a significance of 0.67 and 0.70, according to the measurement scale. The score of the instrument qualifies it as high or acceptable. Therefore, it is resolved that it is valid and can be applied to the study population.

The distribution of items in the ECMA scale of knowledge of contraceptive methods, divides the instrument into dimensions: with a minimum score (pm), and a maximum score (pM), which integrates the indicator, its objective is to know the concepts that the student has, made up of questions 1, 2, 3, 4, 5, 6 and 7, pm. 0 and pM. 7.

Integrate the indicator importance of knowledge: with the objective of knowing other benefits of using contraceptives, with questions: 8, 9 and 10, with pm 0 and pM 3, the indicator type of family planning methods that exist: has the purpose of determining which are the most known by the students, 11, 12, 13, 14 and 15 with pm. 0 and pM 5. The last indicator frequency of use: aims to show the correct way of using the different contraceptive methods, 16, 17, 18, 19, 20 and 21 with pm. 0 and pM 6.

The evaluation of the indicators was determined through statistical indexes, on a scale of 0 to 21, classifying 0 to 5 as low, 6 to 11 as medium and 12 to 21 as high, for the general variable of knowledge of contraceptive methods: the lower the score, the lower the knowledge.

Procedure

This research arises from the problem of school dropout related to early pregnancies among adolescents in the community of El Nigromante, since year after year the number of students who graduate from the Telebachillerato is lower than those who entered. Young people today begin their active sexual life at a very young age, sometimes without using any contraceptive method, either due to lack of knowledge or simply because they believe that there is no consequence for this type of behavior.

Subsequently, the research began in the educational experience, Receptional Experience, in charge of Dr. Blanca Flor Fernandez, where it was determined that the study would belong to the Academic Body Human Development-Veracruz with key: UV-275, led by Dr. Claudia Beatriz Enriquez Hernandez, inserted in the line of generation and application of knowledge (LGAC-1), Health and Education for Human Development, the project "Sexuality and Reproduction" in charge of Dr. Blanca Flor Fernandez.

Once the relevance of the study was evaluated by the Ethics and Research Committee of the School of Nursing, Veracruz Region, Dr. Javier Salazar Mendoza was assigned as project director.

The activities that were carried out were the construction of the project to be implemented, carrying out a documentary review of the subject, then the problem was posed, along with the general and specific objectives, as well as the research question, it should be noted that the study is based on the health promotion model of Nola J. Pender.

From this, the construction of the theoretical-referential framework and methodology began. Also, the instrument that was applied was selected in order to determine the level of knowledge of contraceptive methods among adolescents in a public high school, supported by the informed consent at the time of applying the survey to the students.

Once the design of the study was constructed, the competent authorities were asked to approve the development of the research at the school, explaining the objective of the study and its purpose. Once they gave their consent, the work proceeded, using the structured interview technique and the method was a previously elaborated instrument, obtaining the results that are presented in Chapter VI.

Once the information was obtained through the application of the instrument, it was analyzed in a statistical package (SPSS Inc, 2006), processing and presenting the results in the Microsoft Office package in the Windows operating system, for assimilation and interpretation. The purpose of this study is to identify knowledge deficiencies and to develop strategies and interventions to strengthen this component.

Analysis strategies

The Statistical Package for the Social Sciences (SPSS) version 23 for Windows was used to analyze the data, and Microsoft Office 2013 (Microsoft, 2015) was also used, with the following programs: Excel, Word and PowerPoint. Similarly, descriptive statistics such as percentages, frequency, mean, median and mode were implemented, for the reliability of the instruments, Cronbach's Alpha model was used.

Presentation of results

For the presentation and delivery of the final report, Microsoft Office (Microsoft, 2015) was used, graphs were constructed in Excel and tables were edited, and the written document was elaborated, edited and integrated in Word.

To present the results of the study in the forum of the Receptional Experience, use was made of the Power Point program, ensuring the correct visualization and understanding of the attendees, the bibliographic references and file editing, responded to the guidelines of the American Psychological Association (Viveros, 2010).

Ethical considerations

In order to guide the development of the project, safeguarding the integrity of the participants and the proper handling of the information, the Political Constitution of the United Mexican States was consulted: Article 4, third paragraph, which states that everyone has the right to health protection.

The Law will define the bases and modalities for access to health services and will establish the concurrence of the Federation and the federative entities in matters of general health, in accordance with the provisions of section XVI of article 73.

On the other hand, a determining factor for obtaining truthful and assertive data was the participation of the students by answering the instrument responsibly , ensuring the privacy of the data provided, a procedure carried out based on the stipulations of the General Health Law, in the section on research with human beings (Secretaría de Gobernación 2012), and the Mexican Official Standard NOM-012-SSA3-2012.

That establishes the criteria for the execution of research projects for health in human beings (DOF, 2012).

Likewise, the general provisions of the regulations of the General Health Law on Health Research were taken up. According to what was indicated in the second title, Chapter 1, Article 13, in this process, the criterion of respect for the dignity and protection of the rights and welfare of the subject of the study prevailed.

Individuality and anonymity were protected with respect to the provisions of Title Two, Chapter 1, Article 16, since the instrument did not include personal data or information that could lead to the identification of participants.

In order to comply with the provisions of Title Two, Chapter 1, Article 17, Section 1, this research is considered risk-free, since no intervention or intentional modification was made in the study variables: physiological, psychological or social variables of the participating individuals.

On the other hand, in order to comply with the provisions of Article 21, Sections I, IV, VI, and VII, a clear and complete explanation was provided regarding the justification and the freedom to withdraw from the investigation when deemed pertinent.

Subsequently, authorization was requested from the persons responsible for the educational institution, by means of an official letter issued by the management of the Orizaba School of Nursing, which was delivered by those responsible for the project, and at that time the working groups with whom contact would be made were determined. According to the day assigned in the classrooms where the students were, the project was presented and the signature of the informed consent was requested, in order to respond to the provisions of Title Two, Chapter 1, Article 20.

Another ethical reference for this project was the endorsement of the Code of Nursing Ethics (CIE, 1953), taking up the first axis; The Nurse and the People, where it is established that professionals must ensure an environment of respect, provide the individual with sufficient information to support the consent given to care and related treatments, maintaining confidentiality of all data obtained and using discretion when sharing it.

Likewise, axis three was observed; The Nurse and the Profession, which exposes the implementation of applying acceptable standards in clinical practice, management, research and nursing education, actively contributing to the development of a core of professional knowledge based on research (CIE, 1953).

Finally, this declaration states that in all biomedical research involving human beings, a clear balance must be established between the benefits to be obtained compared to the risks, safeguarding the integrity of individuals, avoiding at all costs causing any harm to the person and their environment, providing them with the knowledge and freedom to abandon the study at the moment they decide to do so (CONAMED, 2008).

Chapter V

Results of the study

MCE. Conzatti Hernández María Esperanza
Dr. Rodríguez Muñoz Ivett
Dr. Contreras Miranda María de Jesús
Dr. Javier Salazar Mendoza
Dr. Castellanos Contreras Edith MCE.
Cabrera Martínez Margarita

The statistical program Statistical Package for the Social Sciences (SPSS, Inc, 2006), version 23 for Windows, was used to analyze the information, creating a database where the instruments were entered, after validation and review of the complete and correct filling of the data.

The analysis plan was integrated by descriptive statistics (Celis & Labrada, 2014), frequency, percentages, measures of central tendency: mean, median, mode, standard deviation, minimum and maximum (Orellana, 2001).

Reliability of the instrument

The internal consistency of the instrument was with the Cronbach's Alpha Reliability scale (García, González & Jornet, 2010), according to Hernández et al. (2014), a result was obtained that ensured the choice of a correct level to evaluate the dependent variable: knowledge of contraceptive methods obtained in the study (Table 1).

Table 1
Reliability of the instrument

InstrumentVariable	**Items**	**Model**	**Reliability**
ECMA Knowledge of methods contraceptives	21	Cronbach's Alpha	0.679

Note: Source: **ECMA:** Contraceptive Methods Knowledge Level Survey (Aranda et al., 2017).

Analysis and interpretation

Table 2
Age and religion by sex of the population

	Sex			
Age	**Female** (*n=29*)		**Male** (*n=24*)	
	f	**%**	**f**	**%**

15 years	4	7.5	4	7.5
16 years old	11	20.8	9	17.0
17 years	5	9.4	5	9.4
18 years old	9	17.0	3	5.7
19 years old	0	0	1	1.9
20 years	0	0	1	1.9
21 years old	0	0	1	1.9
Total	**29**	**54.7%**	**24**	**45.3%**
Religion				
Catholic	28	52.8	20	37.7
Christian	1	1.9	1	1.9
Atheist	0	0	3	5.7
Total	**29**	**54.7%**	**24**	**45.3%**

Note: Source: General data identification card.

Table 2 refers to the sex, age and religion of the students of the Telebachillerato El Nigromante, in relation to the first variable (sex), the female predominated (54.7%), while 45.3% are male, that is, there is a population difference where women exceeded with 9.4%. In terms of age, those who stood out were those individuals aged 16 years (37.8%), 20.8% those aged 17.0%, 18 years 22.7%, and 17 years 18.8%, it should be noted that 20.7% are between 15, 19, 20 and 21.

The analysis of the dispersion measures showed a mean of 16.7+1.3, minimum 15 and maximum 21, median and mode 16, determining that the ranges identified are in accordance with the level of study completed. Of 53 students on the campus, 48 of them reported belonging to the Catholic religion (90.5%), followed by atheists (5.7%), while only 3.8% said they were Christian.

Table 3

Semester, number of siblings and location by sex

Semester	**Sex**			
	Female (*n=29*)		**Male** (*n=24*)	
	f	**%**	**f**	**%**
Second	9	17.0	12	22.6
Fourth	9	17.0	7	13.2
Sixth	11	20.8	5	9.4
Total	**29**	**54.7%**	**24**	**45.3%**
Number of siblings				

1 a 3	17	32.0	15	28.3
4 a 6	10	18.9	7	13.2
7 a 13	2	3.8	2	3.8
Total	**29**	**54.7%**	**24**	**45.3%**
Place in your siblings				
1 a 3	22	41.5	21	39.5
4 a 6	5	9.4	1	1.9
7 a 13	2	3.8	2	3.8
Total	**29**	**54.7%**	**24**	**45.3%**
Note: Source: Data identification card.				

The period that the students are studying, as well as the number of siblings they have and the place of members they occupy is shown in Table 3. In the second semester, the largest population is found with 39.6%, while the fourth and sixth semesters represent 30.2%, each group, showing a range of 9.4% between students who enter high school and those who remain and complete their studies.

In terms of the number of siblings, responses ranged from one to 13, with 26.4% having two, being the most frequent, followed by one, three and five (52.7%) of the total, which means that more than half belong to families with several members. The other 20.9% have four, six, seven, eight and 13 siblings.

Similarly, we surveyed the place they occupy among their siblings, having as a result an order from highest to lowest; the first 50.9%, second 18.8%, third 11.3%, fourth and seventh with 5.7% each. Likewise, it is concluded that most of the students are from the first generation of children, this can be beneficial for them since they have the opportunity to meet their needs in a more complete way, however, the remaining 7.6% are those who integrate the fifth to thirteenth place, this affects their overall performance since they are prone to situations of disinterest.

Table 4

Average, scholarship and type

	Sex			
Average	**Female** (*n=29*)		**Male** (*n=24*)	
	f	**%**	**f**	**%**
Less than 5.9	0	0	1	1.9
6.0 a 6.5	2	3.8	3	5.7
6.6 a 7.0	8	15.1	3	5.7
7.1 a 7.5	4	7.5	9	17.0
7.6 a 8.0	9	17.0	3	5.7

8.1 a 8.5	3	5.7	2	3.8
8.6 a 9.0	2	3.8	2	3.8
9.6 a 10	1	1.9	1	1.9
Total	**29**	**54.7%**	**24**	**45.3%**
Scholarship				
Yes	19	35.8	10	18.9
No	10	18.9	14	26.4
Total	**29**	**54.7%**	**24**	**45.3%**
Type of scholarship				
Prospera	19	35.8	10	18.9
I do not have	10	18.9	14	26.4
Total	**29**	**54.7%**	**24**	**45.3%**

Note: Source: Data identification card.

Bearing in mind that the community of El Nigromante has the Prospera program, which provides economic support to low-income families so that they can cover expenses and encourage young people to continue studying, Table 4 was prepared in order to obtain a precise result.

The average reflected is that obtained up to the previous semester (first, third and fifth), with 7.1 to 7.5 being the most frequent range (24.5%), categorized as poor academic performance, while 39.8% of the population obtained acceptable figures (7.6-8.0, 8.1-8.5 and 8.6-9.0). It is worth noting that only two people have an outstanding quotient of 9.6 to 10, while 1.9% had a failing grade of less than 5.9.

Likewise, it is shown that 54.7% have a scholarship, which is more than half of the population, while the remaining 45.3% do not receive any support from the government or public organizations. Despite the fact that the highest percentage has an income, the others (54.7%), with no help, are still an alarming number since there is only a range of 9.4% difference.

When expressing what type of scholarship the Telebachillerato students have, the answer with the highest percentage was the PROSPERA option (54.7%), this means that 100% enjoy it, which is the only one provided by the community of El Nigromante and it is not for their academic abilities, that is, the average is not a trigger to obtain it, however, it is not reflected in their being a student, since they know the conditions for it.

Table 5

Concepts: definition, use, utilization, use and effects of contraceptive methods

Definition of contraceptive methods	Sex

	Female (*n=29*)		Male (*n=24*)	
	f	%	f	%
Prevent pregnancies	13	24.5	5	9.4
Used at any time	0	0	2	3.8
Protect against STDs*.	16	30.2	17	32.1
Total	**29**	**54.7%**	**24**	**45.3%**
Who can use them				
Adults only	2	3.8	2	3.8
Sexually active people	27	50.9	22	41.5
Total	**29**	**54.7%**	**24**	**45.3%**
If you do not use the methods what happens				
Pregnancy	3	5.7	3	5.7
Contagion of STIs**.	5	9.4	8	15.1
Decreases effectiveness	0	0	3	5.7
All of the above	21	39.6	10	18.9
Total	**29**	**54.7%**	**24**	**45.3%**
Method with fewer side effects				
Morning after pill	11	20.8	10	18.9
Copper T	12	22.6	8	15.1
Breastfeeding	2	3.8	4	7.5
Spermicides	4	7.5	2	3.8
Total	**29**	**54.7%**	**24**	**45.3%**

Note: Source: Survey of Level of Knowledge of Methods Contraceptives (Aranda et al., 2017). STD*: Sexually Transmitted Diseases, STI**: Sexually Transmitted Infections.

Table 5, integrates the concepts of utilization, use and effects, 33.9% of the students believe that contraceptive methods only prevent pregnancies, while 62.3% are aware that they also protect against sexually transmitted diseases, however, the remaining 3.8% assume that they are used at any time without knowing what their benefits or consequences are.

It should be noted that 92.4% know that the use of family planning methods is intended for the entire sexually active population and 7.6% state that they are only for adults, however, more than half (58.5%) determine that not using contraceptives is high risk, since there may be different consequences, such as unwanted pregnancies, infection of sexually transmitted infections, among others.

On the other hand, it is alarming that only 11.3% of the students know that breastfeeding is the method with the least side effects, while the other 88.7% do not.

Table 6

Concepts: menstruation, breastfeeding, sexual relations and methods.

Method to avoid pregnancy	Sex			
	Female (*n=29*)		Male (*n=24*)	
	f	%	f	%
Condom	12	22.6	14	26.4
Copper T	8	15.1	1	1.9
Spermicides	3	5.7	1	1.9
Vasectomy	6	11.3	8	15.4
Total	**29**	**54.7%**	**24**	**45.3%**
The breastfeeding method requires				
Breastfeeding	16	30.2	11	20.8
Being pregnant	8	15.1	5	9.4
Consumption of hormone pills	2	3.8	3	5.7
Start on the first day of menstruation	3	5.7	5	9.4
Total	**29**	**54.7%**	**24**	**45.3%**
Method consisting of not having sexual intercourse on fertile days				
Diaphragm	6	11.3	5	9.4
Spermicide	0	0	2	3.8
Copper T	1	1.9	0	0
Rhythm method	22	41.5	17	32.1
Total	**29**	**54.7%**	**24**	**45.3%**

Note: Source: Survey of Level of Knowledge of Methods Contraceptives (Aranda et al., 2017).

When evaluating the concept of contraceptive methods in Table 6, 49% recognize the condom as the best method to avoid pregnancy, but the highest percentage (51%) state that there are others with greater effectiveness, being in the wrong knowledge.

On the other hand, 51% do know what the breastfeeding method consists of, but the remaining 49% have vague knowledge about it. The rhythm method lies in not having sexual relations during fertile days, as 73.6% of the students affirm.

Table 7
Importance of your knowledge

Sex				
Benefits of barrier methods of contraception	**Female** (*n=29*)		**Male** (*n=24*)	
	f	**%**	**f**	**%**
Are permanent	1	1.9	0	0
No fattening	1	1.9	1	1.9
Prevents STIs*.	22	41.5	19	35.8
They are long-lasting	5	9.4	4	7.5
Total	**29**	**54.7%**	**24**	**45.3%**
Contraceptive method that protects against STIs				
Condom	23	43.4	21	39.6
Diaphragm	1	1.9	3	5.7
Morning after pill	5	9.4	0	0
Total	**29**	**54.7%**	**24**	**45.3%**
Who do you consult for contraceptive use?				
Experienced friends	0	0	1	1.9
Specialist	28	52.8	21	39.6
Family	1	1.9	0	0
Nobody, I read or heard it somewhere.	0	0	2	3.8
Total	**29**	**54.7%**	**24**	**45.3%**

Note: Source: Survey of Level of Knowledge of Methods Contraceptives (Aranda et al., 2017), STIs*: Sexually Transmitted Infections.

Regarding the importance of knowledge of contraceptive methods (Table 7), 77.3% agree that in addition to preventing unwanted pregnancy, another important benefit of family planning methods is that they prevent the spread of sexually transmitted infections. Similarly, 83% affirm that condoms are the only method that protects against STIs, while 17% do not know this.

The majority of students (92.4%) say that it is important to consult a specialist on the use of contraceptive methods; however, the remaining 7.6% believe that any media can help them to make good use of contraceptive methods.

Table 8
Use of existing contraceptive methods

Method that is not permanent _	Female (*n=29*)		Male (*n=24*)	
	f	**%**	**f**	**%**
Copper T	7	13.2	9	17.0
Tubal ligation	7	13.2	6	11.3
Vasectomy	7	13.2	2	3.8
All of the above	8	15.1	7	13.2
Total	**29**	**54.7%**	**24**	**45.3%**
The female condom is a condom type method.				
Sterilization	2	3.8	3	5.7
Barrier	13	24.5	17	32.1
Chemist	9	17.0	2	3.8
Permanent	5	9.4	2	3.8
Total	**29**	**54.7%**	**24**	**45.3%**
Pace method of what type it is				
Chemist	5	9.4	0	0
Sterilization	3	5.7	3	5.7
Natural	20	37.7	21	39.6
Permanent	1	1.9	0	0
Total	**29**	**54.7%**	**24**	**45.3%**

Note: Source: Survey of Level of Knowledge of Methods Contraceptives (Aranda et al., 2017).

Table 8 refers to the different types of contraceptive methods that exist. 30.2% of the students state that the copper T is not a permanent contraceptive method; however, 41.5% affirm that vasectomy and tubal ligation are not permanent contraceptive methods either. Lastly, the remaining 28.3% of the students stated that the three methods mentioned above are definitive.

The female condom is a barrier type of contraceptive, as stated by 56.6% of the population. Seventy-seven percent (77.3%) mention that the rhythm method is of the natural type and only 22.7% of adolescents do not identify it.

Table 9

Use of contraceptive methods in stock

Method used by women of child-bearing age	Female (*n=29*)		Male (*n=24*)	
	f	**%**	**f**	**%**
Birth control pills	11	20.8	2	3.8
Rhythm method	3	5.7	3	5.7
Female condom	4	7.5	11	20.8
All of the above	11	20.8	8	15.1
Total	**29**	**54.7%**	**24**	**45.3%**
Classification of injectable contraceptive methods				
Permanent	2	3.8	3	5.7
Barrier	5	9.4	4	7.5
Effective against STIs	5	9.4	0	0
Hormonal	17	32.1	17	32.1
Total	**29**	**54.7%**	**24**	**45.3%**

Note: Source: Survey of Level of Knowledge of Methods Contraceptives (Aranda et al., 2017), STIs*: Sexually Transmitted Infections.

Table 9 integrates the use of contraceptive methods in existence, where a minority percentage (35.9%), believes that women of childbearing age can use different contraceptives such as: pills, rhythm method and condom, therefore the remaining 64.1% mentions that they only use one type. As for injectable contraceptives, 62.2% confirm that they are for hormonal use, but 37.8% do not distinguish their classification.

Table 10

Frequency of use of methods

The morning-after pill should be	Female (*n=29*)		Male (*n=24*)	
	f	**%**	**f**	**%**
Take every day	0	0	1	1.9
Use after unprotected intercourse	25	47.2	21	39.6
To be used a maximum of 10 times a year	2	3.8	2	3.8
Use weekly	2	3.8	0	0
Total	**29**	**54.7%**	**24**	**45.3%**
To be effective, contraceptive pills must be taken as follows				
After menstruation	7	13.2	4	7.5

Before menstruation	11	20.8	10	18.9
First day of menstrual period	5	9.4	4	7.5
Last day of menstrual period	6	11.3	6	11.3
Total	**29**	**54.7%**	**24**	**45.3%**
When injectables are applied				
Each month	2	3.8	2	3.8
Every 2 months	5	9.4	3	5.7
Every 3 months	3	5.7	3	5.7
Monthly and quarterly	19	35.8	16	30.2
Total	**29**	**54.7%**	**24**	**45.3%**
Condom use				
Only once	28	52.8	23	43.4
Twice, with the same person	0	0	1	1.9
Maximum three times	1	1.9	0	0
Total	**29**	**54.7%**	**24**	**45.3%**

Note: Source: Survey of Level of Knowledge of Methods Contraceptives (Aranda et al., 2017).

When evaluating the frequency of method use (Table 10), the majority (86.8%) stated that the morning-after pill should only be taken after unprotected sexual intercourse; the other 13.2% did not know the appropriate time to take the pill.

Injectables can be administered monthly and quarterly, according to 66% of high school students, while 34% say that they should only be administered monthly, bimonthly or quarterly. Ninety-six percent of the population affirms that condoms should be used only once, since they are not reusable.

Table 11

Use of contraceptive methods in frequency

Condoms at the moment of maximum safety	**Female** (*n=29*)		**Male** (*n=24*)	
	f	**%**	**f**	**%**
Initiation of the sexual act	4	7.5	5	9.4
Before sexual intercourse	23	43.4	18	34.0
We put it on before ejaculating.	2	3.8	1	1.9
Total	**29**	**54.7%**	**24**	**45.3%**

Timing of the morning-after or emergency pill				
10 minutes before intercourse	2	3.8	2	3.8
1 hour before intercourse	3	5.7	1	1.9
The following day	10	18.9	9	17.0
72 hours after sexual intercourse	14	26.4	12	22.6
Total	**29**	**54.7%**	**24**	**45.3%**

Note: Source: Survey of Level of Knowledge of Methods Contraceptives (Aranda et al., 2017).

In Table 11, which describes the frequency of use of conceptive methods, in order for condoms to be safer, they should be used before initiating sexual intercourse, according to 77.4% of the students; on the other hand, the morning after pill or emergency pill should be taken as soon as possible after sexual intercourse (maximum 72 hours later), according to 49% of the students.

Table 12

Knowledge classification

Level	f	%
Definition		
Under	3	5.7
Medium	29	54.7
High	21	39.6
Total	**53**	**100%**
Importance		
Under	5	9.4
Medium	14	26.4
High	34	64.2
Total	**53**	**100%**
Type		
Under	12	22.6
Medium	28	52.8
High	13	24.5
Total	**53**	**100%**
Frequency		

Under	0	0
Medium	17	32.1
High	36	67.9
Total	**53**	**100%**

Note: Source: Contraceptive Methods Knowledge Level Survey (Aranda et al., 2017).

The Survey of Level of Knowledge of Contraceptive Methods (ECMA), by Aranda et al. (2017), is integrated by four dimensions: concept, importance, type, and frequency. From the above information, Table 12 was made to determine the knowledge by dimension that the students of Telebachillerato El Nigromante have about contraceptive methods.

In terms of general concepts, 54.7% have a medium and low knowledge (5.7%), adding the two values, it is determined that 60.4% are not theoretically clear about the definition of these concepts, since only 39.6% do have a direct relationship with the sources of information they have, that is, they prefer to do it with a friend or a peer, although 94.3% stated that a specialist is the ideal person to start using the methods (Table 7).

In relation to the importance of their knowledge, 64.2% obtained a high level, which is of vital risk, since more than half of the population is aware that using some type of contraceptive methods helps them to lead a healthy sexually active life.

However, 26.4% have a medium level, an acceptable percentage because they know the problems involved in not protecting themselves, and therefore do not apply it when having sex. Finally, 9.4% do not consider this to be valuable, since their results were low.

Regarding the different contraceptive methods, the medium level had the highest percentage (52.85%), followed by high knowledge with 24.5%, a range of 1.9% difference, alarming data since almost a quarter of the population studied does not distinguish the types of contraceptive methods that exist, exposing them to potential risks, since having it clear, their choice is wrong, not so for the low level (22.6%), which does carry it out. Finally, in the dimension of frequency of use, the results are better than the previous sections, since no student presented low knowledge and 100% were divided between medium (32.1%) and high (67.9%), being the highest percentage, which shows that the majority of students who are already sexually active use a contraceptive method (Table 12).

Table 13

General knowledge

Knowledge level		
Level	**f**	%
Under	0	0
Medium	13	24.5
High	40	75.5
Total	**53**	**100%**

Note: Source: Contraceptive Methods Knowledge Level Survey (Aranda et al., 2017).

In order to test the hypothesis H_1: the level of knowledge of contraceptive methods among adolescents in the Telebachillerato is low, because sociodemographic characteristics are involved, Table 13 shows the knowledge in general, i.e., the four dimensions of analysis were integrated and a total percentage was obtained.

The final result is favorable, since no one obtained low knowledge, 24.5% is medium, while the high level was the highest percentage with 75.5%, being slightly more than three quarters of the population (an outstanding figure).

With the above, the null hypothesis H_0 is approved: the level of knowledge of contraceptive methods that the Telebachillerato adolescents have is high, because sociodemographic characteristics do not intervene, although it should be noted that the dimensions of: definition (5.7%, lower), importance (9.4%, low), and type (22.6%, low) should be reinforced, since this will help the total number of students to clarify their ideas and make better decisions.

Final considerations

Dr. Méndez Cordero Ernestina
ME. López Ocampo Miguel Ángel
LE. Carral Hernández Brenda Dr. Castellanos Contreras Edith Dr. Javier Salazar Mendoza ESS. Cuervo Pablo Gabriela Berenice

Discussion

Contraceptive methods are substances, objects or procedures used by men and women, preventing unplanned pregnancy, spacing births of children or stopping having children. They help individuals and couples to conceive the number of children they want, at the time they so decide and when they feel more prepared for it, (WHO, 2018). They are also used to prevent sexually transmitted infections.

On the other hand, WHO (2018), defines adolescence as the period of growth and humanistic development that occurs after childhood and before adulthood, between the ages of 10 and 19 years. It is one of the most important transitional stages in the life of the human being, characterized by an accelerated pace of evolution and change.

Many changes have occurred during the past century in relation to this life cycle, in particular the earlier onset of puberty, the postponement of marriage, urbanization, the globalization of communication and the evolution of sexual attitudes and practices.

The population studied consisted of 54.7% women and 45.3% men, coinciding with Aranda et al. (2017), Vargas et al. (2016), Jiménez et al. (2016), Sánchez et al. (2015) and Moreno and Rangel (2012), determining that it is women who make up the largest number of the sample and it is they who provide information on contraceptive methods.

Vargas et al. (2016), In their research on the knowledge and use of contraceptive methods in students of the N°2 high school in the City of Tulancingo de Bravo, they obtained an average general age of 16 years, 54% of the participants were between 15 and 16 years old, coinciding with this study, since most of the students are 16 years old (37.8%) and the average is 16.

On the other hand, Sánchez et al. (2015), in their article Knowledge and use of contraceptive methods among adolescents in a health center, confirms that the male condom is the most known method (100%), followed by oral hormonal methods (87%) and the female condom (85.8%). Thus, of the 120 adolescents, 117 (97.5%) had received information on how to use contraceptive methods, the sources of information coming from teachers (37.5) and health personnel (31.7%).

The results contrast with the present, since only 92.4% of the population prefers to receive information directly from a specialist in order to make better use of the contraceptive methods available. On the other hand, the morning after pill is one of the most known methods (86.8%), followed by the condom (83%), which also protects against sexually transmitted infections and is therefore one of the most used by adolescents.

In 2017 Aranda, Hualpa, Vicente and Millones established the level of knowledge about contraceptive methods in adolescents in secondary education in Lo Olivos, Peru where it shows the highest percentage in the medium level of knowledge with 51.4%, followed by the high level with 47% and the lowest percentage the low level with 9.2%.

These figures agree with the results of this study, since 75.5%, had medium knowledge and 24.5%, in the same way as Jimenez et al. (2016), where 64.7% were medium and 9.4% high and contrasting with Sanchez et al. (2015), who assured that 100%, know contraceptive methods, Vargas et al. (2016), where 100%, had high knowledge, as well as Moreno and Rangel (2012).

Regarding the theoretical discussion with the Health Promotion Model (Pender, et al., 1998), which states that the theory identifies cognitive-perceptual factors in the individual, resulting in participation in health-promoting behaviors, when there is a guideline for action, in this study it was determined that the total population has the intention to participate in care to increase knowledge in the use of contraceptive methods.

After the data collection, they were informed and detailed the consequences of not using any contraceptive method as protection, that is, they were encouraged to participate in the adoption of favorable behaviors and that this was transmitted to others, the total population expressed interest for a change, in order to ingest and verify what is mentioned in the Health Promotion Model (MPS), which is based on the education of people, how to take care of themselves and lead a healthy life, promoting it, since it is paramount, before the care.

Pender et al (1998), in the MPS, cites four paradigms, from which the person was taken, evaluating their sociodemographic characteristics, use and knowledge of contraceptive methods, as well as health problems and limitations.

On the other hand, in Pender's Health Promotion Model, he states that the objective or responsibility of every nursing professional is to provide health care, since it is the basis of any reform plan for such citizens, and the nurse is the main agent in charge of motivating users to maintain their personal health.

In developing this research project and after analyzing the results compared with the MPS rationale, the importance of carrying out interventions in these population groups was determined, in order to strengthen knowledge and beliefs and thus have a greater impact on the issue of adolescent sexuality.

The importance of promoting an optimal state of health by putting preventive actions first. As cited by Pender et al. (1998), is of great interest, given that the factors that influence decision making and the actions taken to prevent the disease were identified, therefore, it is confirmed that the Health Promotion Model is an imminent basis and foundation for nursing professionals, given that, the determinants of health promotion and lifestyles are divided into cognitive-perceptual factors and from these, it was possible to induce the population to behaviors and behaviors through decisions and behaviors that favor health, in order to modify these factors.

This allowed the students to reflect and adopt a responsible promoting behavior in the acquisition of knowledge and modulation of beliefs.

The use and application of Pender's Health Promotion Model in this project was a fundamental basis as an integrating framework for the assessment of knowledge and behaviors, as well as the explanation of the relationships between the factors that are believed to influence changes in health behavior (Giraldo, 2010). In addition, carrying out projects with a quantitative approach allows analyzing the experiences through life histories and determining not only the response, but also the impact and perceiving the damage that has been caused in the affective and physical aspects.

Therefore, it is important to determine the continuous use and application of the MPS, since this helps the nursing professional to be prepared with fundamental tools to act at any time, specifically in adolescent sexuality.

Conclusion

Knowledge of contraceptive methods in adolescents is a topic of great importance nowadays, since it is now common for young minors to become pregnant because of initiating unprotected sex, this leads to act rashly as it is the school drop or perform an abortion with the possibility of attracting subsequent consequences, it should be noted that also prevent STIs. Also, having a high level of knowledge about this problem will help to make good decisions regarding the sexual health of students.

The first specific objective, to characterize the sociodemographic data of the population, showed that the age of the participants ranged from 15 to 21 years, with a mean of 16.72, a median of 16 and a mode of 16. There were a total of 53 students, of whom the female sex predominated (54.7%) over the male sex (45.3%), and the Catholic religion was more frequent (90.5%).

With regard to the second objective, to evaluate the students' concept of contraceptive methods, it was found that 39.6% have a clear theoretical definition of contraceptive methods, while the other 60.4% have insufficient knowledge. It is important to highlight that the majority of students (62.3%) are aware that contraceptive methods not only prevent pregnancies, but also protect against sexually transmitted diseases.

Regarding the third specific objective, to identify the contraceptive methods of greatest selection and use in the study population, the results were favorable since no one obtained a low level, while 67.9% stated that they were clear about what type of method to use and when, but 32.1% did not know.

The morning-after pill is one of the most widely known and sometimes misused methods, however, the majority of high school students (86.8%) know when it is appropriate to take this contraceptive, but the remaining 13.2% believe that they can take it whenever they want without knowing the side effects it may have.

Regarding the fourth specific objective: to classify the knowledge and importance of contraceptive methods among adolescents in the Telebachillerato, 83% agree that condoms are the only method that protects against sexually transmitted diseases.

On the other hand, 7.6% believe that any means of dissemination is adequate to provide guidance on the proper use of contraceptive methods; however, the majority (92.4%) state that it is vitally important to consult a specialist on the use of contraceptive methods. Similarly, it is reflected that not all students identify the different types of contraceptives that exist, confusing barrier methods with permanent ones, but 77.3% know how to classify the natural rhythm method.

Given the working hypothesis (H1): the level of knowledge of contraceptive methods among adolescents in the Telebachillerato El Nigromante, Veracruz, is low because sociodemographic characteristics are involved, a table was made in order to test or reject the hypothesis, as a result of this it was obtained that the H0: The level of knowledge of contraceptive methods among adolescents of the Telebachillerato El Nigromante, Veracruz, is high because sociodemographic characteristics do not play a role, since the analysis showed that 75.5% of the population has a high level of knowledge about the topic of study.

While the other 24.5% of adolescents are in the middle level, therefore no one obtained low knowledge about contraceptive methods, speaking of general percentages.

From the above, it is concluded that in the telebachillerato El Nigromante most of the students have a high knowledge, despite this favorable result, it is of vital importance to reinforce certain dimensions in which not everyone scored well, implementing various interventions between teachers, students and health personnel.

Therefore, there is a need to implement effective and efficient nursing interventions, using the proposal of Nola J. Pender's Health Promotion Model, which states that the individual is capable of adopting health-promoting behaviors for the benefit of his or her health, in order to maintain effective health conditions, as long as he or she is stimulated by health professionals highly trained in the subject (Pender et al., 1998).

The final results show the importance of addressing the young population, especially if they are exposed to risks, so other components should be explored in order to reinforce and, together with nursing professionals, implement working groups to address the problem.

Recommendations

To train the nursing staff currently inserted in the work environment, in order to achieve through good information the knowledge of contraceptive methods.

To carry out work related to the studied populations, thus confirming or denying in the future their increased knowledge about contraceptive methods with the expansion of knowledge imparted.

Implement joint actions between the health center and schools, in order to reinforce reproductive health issues and prevent sexually transmitted infections or unwanted pregnancies in adolescents.

To educate students about health issues in order to raise awareness and motivate them to adopt actions in favor of their well-being and quality of life.

Train the school's teaching staff on health topics so that they can inform students about them and thus increase their knowledge of contraceptive methods.

Conduct activities that serve as an evaluation of adolescents (health fairs, class discussions), to determine whether the actions implemented are adequate and favorable to them.

Raise awareness among parents so that they also implement sexuality topics with their children at home.

Implement sexual and reproductive education in schools as an interdisciplinary process.

Bringing together authorities and health centers to organize programs in the community to address sexual health issues in parents and children.

To teach undergraduate nursing students strategies to address health promotion with adolescents.

Bibliographic references

Aranda, X. A., Huallpa, M. E., Vicente, F. L., & Millones, S. G. (2017). *Level of knowledge about contraceptive methods in adolescents of secondary education of the private educational institution Bertrand Rusell, Los Olivos 2015.* (Bachelor's thesis). Retrieved from http://repositorio.uch.edu.pe/bitstream/handle/uch/145/Aranda_XA_Hua llp a_MS_Vicente_Vicente_FL_TENF_2017.pdf?sequence=1&isAllowed=y

Chilean Institute of Reproductive Medicine (ICMER, 2018). *Emergency contraception.* Retrieved from http://icmer.org/wp_ae/informacion- general-2/

National Institute of Statistics and Geography (INEGI, 2016). *Statistics on the occasion of International Youth Day.* Retrieved from http:// www.inegi.org.mx/saladeprensa/aproposito/2016/juventud2016_0.pd

Mosquera, J., & Mateus, J. C. (2003*). Knowledge, attitudes and practices about family planning methods, HIV-AIDS and media use in young people.* Retrieved from: file:///C:/Users/nayel/Docu ments/ Experiencia%20Recepcional/doc.pdf.

World Health Organization. (WHO, 2009). *Adolescent Health Orientation Program for Health Care Providers.* Retrieved from http://new.paho.org/hq/dmdocuments/2009/orientation%20modules%20 WHO.pdf

World Health Organization. (WHO, 2014). *Health for the world's adolescents.* Retrieved from: http://www. who.int/mediacentre/news/rel eases/2014/focus-adolescent-health/en/

Ministry of Public Education (SEP, January 18, 2015). Inicia vida sexual entre 12 y 15 años. *Excélsior newspaper.* Retrieved from http://ww w.excelsior.co m.mx/nacional/2015/ 01/18/1003289

Silva, I. V. (September 16, 2013). Adolescents are slow to use contraceptives. *Periódico Excélsior.* Retrieved from https://www.excelsi or.com.mx/nacional/2013/09/16/918830#view-5.

Aller, J. & Pagés, G. (1998). *Contraceptive methods. Venezuela:* Second edition. Editorial McGraw-Hill, Interamericana.

Aranda, X. A., Huallpa, M. E., Vicente, F. L., & Millones, S. G. (2017). *Level of knowledge about contraceptive methods in adolescents of secondary education of the private educational institution Bertrand Rusell, Los Olivos 2015.* (Bachelor's thesis). Retrieved from http://repositorio.uch.edu.pe/bitstream/handle/uch/145/Aranda_XA_Hua llp a_MS_Vicente_Vicente_FL_TENF_2017.pdf?sequence=1&isAllowed=y

Asociación Mexicana de Agencias de Investigación y Opinión Pública A.C. (AMAI, 2004). *Classification of socioeconomic levels in Mexico according to AMAI.* Retrieved from http://www.fergut.com/clasificacion-de-niveles-socioeconomicos -en-mexico-segun-la-amai/

Ayala, A. J., & Pereira, C. (2014). *Use of contraceptive methods in young people from a gender perspective: a vision from health education.* (Undergraduate thesis, Universidad Autónoma del Estado de México). Retrieved from http://ri.uaemex.mx/bitstream/handle/20.500. 11799/66673/2014%2C%20AYALA%2C%20METODOS%20ANTICONC EPTIVOS-split-merge.pdf?sequence=3&isAllowed=y

Benetti, S. (2011). *Comprehensive training: sexuality.* Retrieved from http://form aci on-integ ral.com.ar/website/?p=17

Casaya, M. (2017). *Knowledge, attitudes and practices of nursing staff on biosafety standards in hemodialysis procedures, Dr. Alejandro Dávila Bolaños military hospital, Managua, Nicaragua.* Retrieved from http://repositorio.unan.edu.ni/ 7912/1/t955.pdf.

National Population Council (CONAPO, 2014). *National Survey of Demographic Dynamics.* Retrieved from http://www.inegi.org.mx/salade prensa/boletines/2015/especiales/especiales2015_07_1.pdf.

National Population Council (CONAPO, 2016). *Sexual and reproductive health situation.* Retrieved from http://www.omm.org.mx/images/ stories/Documentos%20grandes/Situacion_SS_y_R_2016.pdf.

Health Sciences Descriptors. (DeCS, 2018). *Knowledge.* Retrieved from http://decs.bvs.br/cgi-bin/wxis1660.exe/decsserver/

Official Journal of the Federation (2018). *Political Constitution of the United Mexican States of 1917.* Retrieved from http://www.diputados.gob. mx/LeyesBiblio/pdf/1_270818.pdf.

Diario Oficial de la Federación (Official Gazette of the Federation) (2018). *Ley General de Población de 1974.* Retrieved from http://www.diputados.gob.mx/LeyesBiblio/pdf/140_1207 18.pdf

Official Journal of the Federation (DOF, 1993). *Norma Oficial Mexicana, NOM 005-SSA2-1993, De los Servicios de Planificación Familiar (Official Mexican Standard, NOM 005-SSA2-1993, On Family Planning Services).* Retrieved from *http://www.salud.gob.mx/unidades/cdi/nom/005ssa23.h tml*

Official Gazette of the Federation (DOF, 2000). *Law for the protection of the rights of children and adolescents.* Retrieved from https://docs.mexico.justia.com/federales/ley_para_la_proteccion_de_los_derecho s_de _ninas_ninos_ninos_y_adolescentes.pdf

National Health and Nutrition Survey (ENSANUT, 2006). *Final report of results.* Retrieved from http://transparencia.insp.mx/2017/auditorias insp/12701_Resultados_E ncuesta_ENSANUT_MC2016.pdf.

Gabarro, B. D. (2010). *School failure: the unexpected solution of gender and coeducation*. Lleida: Boira Editorial.

Hoffe, O. (2004). *Breve historia ilustrada de la filosofía, El mundo de las ideas*. Barcelona, Spain: Ediciones Península.

Mexican Institute of Social Security (2015). *Family Planning*. Retrieved from http://www.imss.gob.mx/salud-en-linea/planificacion- family

National Institute of Statistics and Geography (INEGI, 2015). *National survey of demographic dynamics 2014.* Retrieved from http://www.inegi.org.mx/saladeprensa/boletines/2015/especiales/especi ales2015_07_1.pdf.

National Institute of Statistics and Geography (INEGI, 2016). *Statistics on the purpose of international youth day.* Retrieved from http://www.inegi.org.mx/saladeprensa/aproposito/2016/juventud2016_0. pd

Jiménez, D. I., Vilchis, E., & Martínez, M. D. (2016). *Level of knowledge about contraceptive methods that students of a Mexiquense high school have (*Bachelor's thesis). Retrieved from http://ri.uaemex.mx/bitstream/handle/20.500.11799/66316/TESIS%20(6)-split-merge.pdf?sequen ce=3

López, F. (2003). *Papyrus Ebers-The most important medical papyrus.* Retrieved from http://egiptologia.org/?page_id=1149

Maier, C. (2017). *5 characteristics of adolescence.* Retrieved from http://www.ehowenespanol.com/5caracteristicasadolescenciainfo_1112 39

Marcos, M. A., (1988). *Pierre Duhem: The philosophy of science in its origins.* Retrieved from http://www.fyl.uva.es/~wfilosof/webMarcos/text os/Duhem_complete_book.pdf

Martos, A. (2009). *Brief history of condoms and contraceptive methods.* Retrieved from www.books.google.com

Moreno, J. N., & Rangel, D. C. (2012). *Knowledge about contraceptive methods in 9th grade students of the U.E. Nuestra Señora de Lourdes, Puerto Ordaz, Bolivar state* (Undergraduate Thesis). Retrieved from http://hdl.handle. net/123456789/2226

World Health Organization. (WHO, 2015). *Trends in Contraceptive Use Worldwide.* Retrieved from http://www.un.org/en/development/desa/ population/publications/pdf/family/trendsContraceptiveUse2015Report.pd f

World Health Organization. (WHO, 2015). *World contraceptive patterns.* Retrieved from http://www.un.org/en/development/desa/popu lation/publ ications/pdf/family/Infochart-World-Contraceptive-Patterns-2015.pdf.

World Health Organization. (WHO, 2016). *Maternal, newborn, child and adolescent health.* Retrieved from http://www.who.int/m aternal _child_adolescent/topics /adolescence/en/

World Health Organization. (WHO, 2018). *Maternal, newborn, child and adolescent health, Adolescent development.* Retrieved from http://www.who.int/maternal_child_adolescent/topics/ad olescence/dev/en

Pan American Health Organization. (2007). *Health in the Americas Vol. 2-Profiles by Country 2007.* Retrieved from https://www.paho.org/cor/inde x.php?option=com_docman&view=download&alias=257-health-in-the-americas-2007-vol-2&category_slug=publications&Itemid=222

Organisation for Economic Co-operation and Development (OECD, 2014). *Education at a glance.* Retrieved from https://www.mecd.gob.es/d ctm/inee/inee/indicadoreseducativos/panorama2014/panorama2014web.pdf ?documentId=0901e72b81b20622

Pérez, P. J (2008). *Definition of: Definition of knowledge.* Retrieved from https://definicion.de/conocimiento/

Ruiz, P. J. (2013). School problems in adolescence. *Revista Pediatría Integral, XVII*(2). Retrieved from https://www.pediatriaintegral. es/numeros-anteriores/publicacion-2013-03/los-problemas-escolares- en-la-adolescencia/

Sánchez, M. C., Dávila, R., & Ponce E. F. (2015). Knowledge and use of contraceptive methods among adolescents in a health center. *Revista atención familiar, 22*(2). doi: 10.1016/S1405-8871(16)30044-X.

Sanyo, S., & Molina, R. (2005). *History of Contraception. Online manual of the Latin American Center for Health and Women.* Retrieved from http.www.www.c elsam.org/home/manual.a sp?cvemanual=7,

SecretaríadeSalud (2005). *LeyGeneraldeSalud.* retrievedfrom http://www.salud.gob.mx/cnts/pdfs/LEY_GENERAL_DE_SALUD.pdf

SecretaríadeSalud .(2015).LeyGeneraldeSalud . Recoveredfrom. https://www.ucol.mx/content/cms/13/file/federal/LEY_GRAL_DE_SALUD .pdf

Semilla, D. F. (2011). *Contemporary philosophy: Auguste Comte, Summary of the modern past.* Retrieved from http://textosfil.blogspot.mx/2011/09/au gusto-comte-sumario-del-pastado.html.

University of Chile (2017). *General characteristics of the BIO- PSYCHO-SOCIAL Development of adolescence*. Retrieved from http://educacionse xual.uchile.cl/index.php/hablando-de-sexo/adolescencia/desarrollo-bio- psico-social-de-la-adolescencia.

Vargas, S., Yunez, E. M., & Ramírez, M. D. (2016). *Evaluation of the knowledge and use of contraceptive methods in high school students №2 of the City of Tulancingo de Bravo, Hidalgo, 2015* (Bachelor's Thesis). Retrieved from http://catalogoinsp.mx/files/tes/ 055185.pdf.

Weiner, B. (1986). *An attributional theory of motivation and emotion*. USA, New York: Springer Verlag.

National Commission of Medical Arbitration (CONAMED, 2008). *Helsinki declaration standards.* Retrieved from http://www.wma.net/es/30publi cations/10policies/b3/17c_en.pdf.

International Council of Nurses (ICN, 1953*). ICN code of ethics for the nursing profession.* Retrieved from http://castellon.sa n.gva.es/documents/4434516/5188103/Codigo+Deontol ogico+CIE.pdf.

Mariner, A., & Raile, M. (2007). *Models and theories in nursing.* Seventh edition. Publisher: Elsevier Science Madrid Spain.

Pender, N. J. (1996). *Health promotion in nursing practice* (3rd ed.). Stamford, CT: Appleton & Lange.

Pender, N. J., Walker, S. N., Sechrist, K. R., & Stromborg, M. F. (1998). *Development and testing of the Health Promotion* Model. *Cardiovascular Nursing, 24*(6), 41-43.

Pender, N. J., Walker, S. N., Stromborg, M.F., & Sechrist, K.R. (2009). *Predicting health-promoting lifestyles in the workplace. Nursing Research. 39*(6). Retrieved from https://www.ncbi.nlm.nih.gov/pub med/2092305

Secretary of the Interior (2012). *Reglamento de la ley general de salud en materia de investigación para la salud.* Retrieved from http://www.salud .gob.mx/ unidades /cdi/nom/compi/rlgsmis.html.

Aranda, X. A., Huallpa, M. E., Vicente, F. L., & Millones, S. G. (2017). *Level of knowledge about contraceptive methods in adolescents of secondary education of the private educational institution Bertrand Rusell, Los Olivos 2015.* (Bachelor's thesis). Retrieved from http://r epositorio.uch.edu.pe/bitstream/handle/uch/145/Aranda_XA_Huallpa_M S S_Vicente_FL_TENF_2017.pdf?sequence=1&isAllowed=y

Canales, F. H., Alvarado, E. L., & Pineda, E. B. (2013). *Metodología de la investigación; Manual para el desarrollo de personal de salud.* Mexico: Limusa.
National Commission of Medical Arbitration (CONAMED, 2008). *Helsinki declaration standards.* Retrieved from http://www.wma.net/es/30publi cations/10policies/b3/17c_en.pdf.

International Council of Nurses (ICN, 1953*). ICN code of ethics for the nursing profession.* Retrieved from http://castellon.sa

n.gva.es/documents/4434516/5188103/Codigo+Deontol ogico+CIE.pdf.
Official Journal of the Federation (DOF, 2012). *Norma Oficial Mexicana NOM- 012-SSA3-2012, Que establece los criterios para la ejecución de proyectos de investigación para la salud en seres humanos.* Retrieved from http://dof.gob.mx/nota_detalle.phpcodigo=5284148&fe cha=04/01/20 13.

Grove, S., Gray, J., & Burns, N. (2016). *Nursing research; Developing evidence-based nursing practice (6ª Edition).* Barcelona, Spain: ELSEVIER.

Microsoft (2015). *Office 2013 quick start guides*. Retrieved from https ://support.office.com/en/article/Office-2013-Quick-start-guides- 4a8aa04a-f7f3-4a4d-823c3dbc4b8672a1?CorrelationId=10bc30cd-bb0a- 4258-a154-5e3cf4d78e1c&ui=esES&rs=esES&ad=ES&ocmsassetID=H A103673669

Ortiz, F. G., & García, M. (2014). *Research methodology; The process and its techniques.* Mexico: LIMUSA.

Polit, D., & Hungler, B. (2000). *Scientific research in the health sciences*. Sixth Edition. Mexico DF: Mc Graw-Hill interamericana.

Secretaria de Gobernación (2012), *Reglamento de la ley general de salud en materia de investigación para la salud.* Retrieved from http://www.salud .gob.mx/ unidades /cdi/nom/compi/rlgsmis.html.

Secretaria de Gobernación (2012), *Reglamento de la Ley General de Salud en Materia de Investigación para la Salud.* Retrieved from http://www.s alud.gob.mx/unidades /cdi/nom/compi/rlgsmis.html.

Secretaria de Gobernación (2012). *Constitución Política De Los Estados Unidos Mexicanos*. Retrieved from http://www.sct.gob.mx/JUR E/doc/cp eum.pdf.

Secretaría de Salud. (2005). *General Health Law*. Retrieved from http://www.salud.gob.mx/cnts/pdfs/LEY_GENERAL_DE_SALUD.pdf

SPSS, Inc. (2006). *Brief guide to SPSS 15.0.* Retrieved from http://www.um.es/ae/soloumu/pdfs/pdfs_manuales_spss/SPSS%20Brief %20Guide%2015.0.pdf.

Tamayo, M. (2014). *El proceso de la investigación científica.* Mexico: LIMUSA.

Viveros, S. (2010). *Publication manual of the American Psychological Association (3ª Edition).* NE. Washington DC: The Modern Handbook.

Aranda, X. A., Huallpa, M. E., Vicente, F. L., & Millones, S. G. (2017). *Level of knowledge about contraceptive methods in adolescents of secondary education of the private educational institution Bertrand Rusell, Los Olivos 2015.* (Bachelor's thesis). Retrieved from http://r epositorio.uch.edu.pe/bitstream/handle/uch/145/Aranda_XA_Huallpa_M S S_Vicente_FL_TENF_2017.pdf?sequence=1&isAllowed=y

Celis, A., & Labrada, V. (2014). *Bioestadística (3ª Edición).* Mexico: El Manual Moderno.

García, R., González, J., & Jornet, J. M. (2010). *SPSS: reliability analysis. Cronbach's alpha.* Retrieved from https://www.uv.es/innomide/spss/SP SS/ SPSS _080 1B.pdf.

Hernández, R., Fernández, C., & Baptista, P. (2014). *Metodología de la investigación (*6th Ed). México D.F., México: Interamericana editores, S.A de C.V.

Orellana, L. (2001). *Estadística descriptiva.* Retrieved from http://www.dm.ub a.ar/materias/estadistica_Q/2011/1/modulo%20descriptiva.pdf.

SPSS, Inc. (2006). *Brief guide to SPSS 15.0.* Retrieved from http://www.um.es/ae/soloumu/pdfs/pdfs_manuales_spss/SPSS%20Brief

%20Guide%2015.0.pdf.

Aranda, X. A., Huallpa, M. E., Vicente, F. L., & Millones, S. G. (2017). *Level of knowledge about contraceptive methods in adolescents of secondary education of the private educational institution Bertrand Rusell, Los Olivos 2015.* (Bachelor's thesis). Retrieved from http://repositorio.uch.edu.pe/bitstream/handle/uch/145/Aranda_XA_Hua llp a_MS_Vicente_Vicente_FL_TENF_2017.pdf?sequence=1&isAllowed=y

Giraldo, F. (2010). The evolutionary theory of knowledge. Colombia. Retrieved from http://www.facso.uchile.cl/publicaciones/moebio/mobile/20/giraldo.html

Moreno, J. N., & Rangel, D. C. (2012). *Knowledge about contraceptive methods in 9th grade students of the U.E. Nuestra Señora de Lourdes, Puerto Ordaz, Bolivar state* (Undergraduate Thesis). Retrieved from http://hdl.handle. net/123456789/2226

Jiménez, D. I., Vilchis, E., & Martínez, M. D. (2016). *Level of knowledge about contraceptive methods that students of a Mexiquense high school have* (Bachelor's thesis). Retrieved from http://ri.uaemex.mx/bitstream/handle/20.500.11799/66316/TESIS%20(6)-split-merge.pdf?sequen ce=3

World Health Organization. (WHO, 2018). *Maternal, newborn, child and adolescent health, Adolescent development.* Retrieved from. http://www.who.int/maternal_child_adolescent/topics/adole scence/dev/en

World Health Organization. (WHO, 2018). Family planning. Retrieved from https://www.who.int/es/news-room/fact-sheets/detail/family-planning-contraception

Pender, N. J., Walker, S. N., Sechrist, K. R., & Stromborg, M. F. (1998). *Development and testing of the Health Promotion* Model. *Cardiovascular Nursing, 24*(6), 41-43.

Sánchez, M. C., Dávila, R., & Ponce E. F. (2015). Knowledge and use of contraceptive methods in adolescents in a health center. *Revista atención familiar, 22*(2). doi: 10.1016/S1405-8871(16)30044-X.

Vargas, S., Yunez, E. M., & Ramírez, M. D. (2016). *Evaluation of the knowledge and use of contraceptive methods in high school students №2 of the City of Tulancingo de Bravo, Hidalgo, 2015* (Bachelor's Thesis). Retrieved from http://catalogoinsp.mx/files/tes/ 055185.pdf.

Annexes

Annex 1. Informed Consent
Universidad Veracruzana
School of Nursing
Veracruz Region
Informed consent

By signing this document, I give my consent to participate voluntarily in the present activity **"Knowledge of contraceptive methods in adolescents of the Telebachillerato El Nigromante, Veracruz"** which is related to my daily life. I consider that the results of this study will be of benefit to improve preventive health programs.

My participation consists of answering some questions and allowing care or procedures to be performed on me that do not put my physical and emotional integrity at risk. Also, I was told that the data I provide will be confidential, without the possibility of individual identification and also that I can stop participating in this research at any time I wish. On the other hand, I authorize those responsible for the research to enter my school career, to obtain true and real data, with this, to provide recommendations to the curriculum of the Bachelor's Degree in Nursing.

Gabriela Berenice Cuervo Pablo, a student of the Bachelor's Degree in Nursing, is conducting the study under the direction of **Dr. Javier Salazar Mendoza,** who is responsible for the research.

Interviewee's signature

Gabriela Berenice Cuervo Pablo **Dr. Javier Salazar Mendoza**

Responsible

Annex 2. Sociodemographic data form
Universidad Veracruzana
School of Nursing
Veracruz Region
Sociodemographic data form

Instructions: The instrument has the following aspects in its structure: it presents 21 items of knowledge of contraceptive methods, divided into four dimensions: A. Concept: general according to WHO. B. Importance: Knowledge of contraceptive methods. C. Type of contraceptive methods that exist. D. Frequency: Of the use of the methods. **Answer in the line and paragraph, placing a circle in the option you consider to be the best**, the information requested, remember that the data provided are confidential and anonymity is kept.

1. **General data**
Age: ___ years **old. Marital status:** ______ **Religion:** ______ **Sex: F** ___ **M** ___

Current semester of study: ________________________________
Number of siblings in your family: __________________________

Place you occupy among your siblings: ______________ **Do you have any type of scholarship? YES** __ **NO** __ **Which one?** ________

Indicate the average you have had during high school, up to the current semester (approximately)

-5.9 6 ___ **.0-6.5 6** _______ **.6-7.0 7**_______ **.1-7.5 7** ________ **.6-8.0** ________
8.1-8.5 8 ___ **.6-9.0 9** _______ **.1-9.5 9**________ **.6-10** ________

Annex 3. Research instrument
Universidad Veracruzana
School of Nursing
Veracruz Region
Research Instrument

A. Dimensions concept

1. What are contraceptive methods?

a) These are methods that can be used without medical indication.
b) They are methods that prevent unwanted pregnancies.
c) These are methods that we can use at any time.
d) They are methods that protect against sexually transmitted diseases.

B. Importance of your knowledge

8. Besides protecting you from pregnancy, what other important benefit do barrier methods of contraception have?

a) Are permanentb) Are not fattening
c) It prevents sexually transmitted infections d) They are long lasting.

C. Type of contraceptive methods available

11. What is NOT a permanent method of contraception?

a) Copper Tb) Tubal ligation
c) Vasectomyd) All of the above

D. Frequency of use of methods

16. The morning after pill is a method of contraception that...

a) It should be taken every day b) It should only be used after having sexual intercourse without contraceptive protection

c) Can be used a maximum of 10 times a year d) Used on a weekly basis

If you are interested in consulting the measuring instrument, please click here.

Aranda, X. A., Huallpa, M. E., Vicente, F. L., & Millones, S. G. (2017). *Level of knowledge about contraceptive methods in adolescents of secondary education of the private educational institution Bertrand Rusell, Los Olivos 2015.* (Bachelor's thesis). Retrieved from http://r positorio.uch.edu.pe/bitstream/handle/uch/145/Aranda_XA_Huallpa_M S S_Vicente_FL_TENF_2017.pdf?sequence=1&isAllowed=y

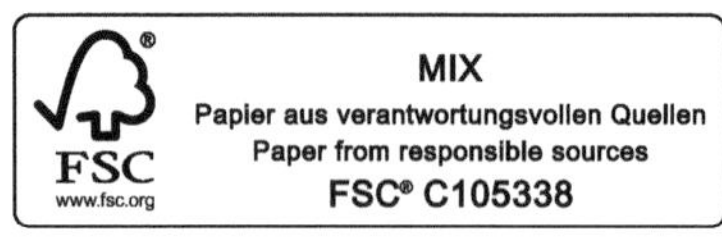

Printed by Books on Demand GmbH, Norderstedt / Germany